Recent Results in Cancer Research 73

Fortschritte der Krebsforschung
Progrès dans les recherches sur le cancer

Thyroid Cancer

Edited by William Duncan

With 58 Figures and 30 Tables

Springer-Verlag
Berlin Heidelberg New York 1980

William Duncan

Department of Radiotherapy,
Western General Hospital, Crewe Road,
GB – Edinburgh EH4 2XU

Sponsored by the Swiss League against Cancer

ISBN-13:978-3-642-81327-6 e-ISBN-13:978-3-642-81325-2
DOI: 10.1007/978-3-642-81325-2

Library of Congress Cataloging in Publication Data. Main entry under title: Thyroid cancer. (Recent results in cancer research; 73) Based on the presentations made at the First Symposium on Clinical Oncology, organized by the Royal College of Radiologists, London, on 26–27 Jan. 1979. Includes bibliographies and index. 1. Thyroid gland-Cancer-Congresses. I. Duncan, William, 1930– II. Series. [DNLM: 1. Thyroid neoplasms-Congresses. W1 RE 106P v. 73/WK270 S988 1979t] RC261.R35 vol. 73 [RC280.T6] 616.99'4s 80-16145 [616.99'444]

2125/3140–5 4 3 2 1 0

Preface

The subject of this publication, thyroid cancer, was the topic chosen for the First Symposium on Clinical Oncology, organized by the Royal College of Radiologists, London, on 26 and 27 January 1979.

The papers collected here are based on the presentations made at that meeting, but have been expanded in most cases to provide a more complete review. Thyroid cancer is an uncommon tumor, but as a result of well-directed collaborative efforts our knowledge of its pathogenesis, natural history, and management has increased enormously in the last decade. Consideration of this progress in our understanding of thyroid cancer well illustrates the main theme to be promoted in this and future symposia, which is the encouragement of a multidisciplinary approach to the solution of the many outstanding problems in clinical oncology. The need is recognized for close and sustained collaboration between clinicians of many speciality groups and research workers of many scientific disciplines, to accelerate further progress in the prevention, early detection, and management of all forms of malignant disease. Thyroid cancer provides an excellent example of the present achievements of such a multidisciplin-

ary approach, where British research and experience have made a contribution that has received world wide recognition. Thyroid cancer, although presenting an uncommon challenge to most clinicians, is of general interest to oncologists, physicians, surgeons, and many non-clinical specialists. Its study has highlighted common principles in clinical oncology: identification of causative factors and reduction of potential hazards; the control of cell proliferation; the importance of histological classification and a sound understanding of surgical pathology; the increasing relevance of tumour marker substances, and the interrelated roles of the many methods of management. Consideration of the evolution of our improved understanding of thyroid cancer may well provide important conceptual leads for other, more common forms of human cancer.
Many years ago, Louis Pasteur offered the opinion that the ultimate reward of a scientist was to see the results of his endeavours applied for the benefit of mankind. It is gratifying that this collection of papers demonstrates in many ways how the results of recent laboratory and clinical research have been shown to be of direct benefit to patients by leading to the establishment of a more rational basis for their management.
It is to be hoped that this publication will at once provide a source of relevant scientific and clinical information on thyroid cancer and a stimulus for further research and evaluation of the many deficiencies in our knowledge that remain to be made good.
My personal thanks must be expressed to distinguished contributors, and especially to those who also participated in the symposium. I have also to record my appreciation of the efforts of my Secretary, Mrs. J. Young, who so ably helped with the organization of the meeting and with the editing and preparation of the manuscripts. A special word of gratitude must go to Mr. Michael Jackson of Springer-Verlag for his helpful, active support, and patient co-operation in the publication of these collected papers.

It is with deep regret that I have to record the death of Dr. G. W. Dolphin last year. His contribution to our understanding of radiation hazards was internationally recognised, and I am proud to be able to include his presentation in this volume.

Edinburgh, 1980 WILLIAM DUNCAN

Contents

M. R. Alderson:
Epidemiology 1

G. W. Dolphin:
Radiation Carcinogenesis 23

D. S. Munro:
Dysplasia and Neoplasia 31

C. J. Edmonds:
Control Mechanism and Stimulation 37

E. D. Williams:
Pathology and Natural History 47

R. Hall, M. Ross, C. S. Teng, and B. Rees Smith:
Immunological Aspects of Thyroid Cancer 56

J. C. Stevenson and C. J. Hillyard:
Tumour Markers 60

M. N. Maisey and S. Ng Tang Fui:
Nuclear Medicine in the Assessment of Thyroid Cancer 68

B. Eddleston:
Radiological Assessment 87

S. Taylor and K. Al-Wattar:
Surgical Management 102

A. W. G. Goolden:
Radiotherapy 112

J. A. Strong:
Medical Management 124

K. E. Halnan:
Perspectives and Prospects 129

Subject Index 139

List of Contributors

M. R. Alderson
Institute of Cancer Research, Sutton (U. K.)

K. Al-Wattar
Hammersmith Hospital, London (U. K.)

G. W. Dolphin
National Radiological Protection Board, Harwell (U. K.)

B. Eddleston
Christie Hospital and Holt Radium Institute, Manchester (U. K.)

C. J. Edmonds
University College Hospital, London (U. K.)

A. W. G. Goolden
Royal Postgraduate Medical School and Hammersmith Hospital, London (U. K.)

R. Hall
Royal Victoria Infirmary, Newcastle-upon-tyne (U. K.)

K. E. Halnan
Royal Postgraduate Medical School and Hammersmith Hospital, London (U. K.)

C. J. Hillyard
Royal Postgraduate Medical School, London (U. K.)

M. N. Maisey
Guy's Hospital, London (U. K.)

D. S. Munro
University of Sheffield and Royal Infirmary, Sheffield (U. K.)

S. Ng Tang Fui
Guy's Hospital,London (U. K.)

B. Rees Smith
Royal Victoria Infirmary, Newcastle-upon-Tyne (U. K.)

W. M. Ross
Royal Victoria Infirmary, Newcastle-upon-Tyne (U. K.)

J. C. Stevenson
Royal Postgraduate Medical School, London (U. K.)

J. A. Strong
University of Edinburgh and Western General Hospital, Edinburgh (U. K.)

S. Taylor
Hammersmith Hospital, London (U. K.)

C. S. Teng
Royal Victoria Infirmary, Newcastle-upon-Tyne (U. K.)

E. D. Williams
Welsh National School of Medicine and University Hospital of Wales, Cardiff (U. K.)

Epidemiology

M. R. Alderson

Division of Epidemiology, Institute of Cancer Research, GB-Sutton, Surrey, SM2 5PX

Introduction

This Chapter begins with a brief review of routine national statistics on the mortality and incidence of thyroid cancer. Such material is often difficult to interpret, due to its inherent errors and biases; a subsection discusses a number of specific problems with these data on thyroid disease. Sections of factors known or suspected to be associated with the development of thyroid cancer then follow. Irradiation is the most clearly documented aetiological factor, and this is considered in detail in Chapter 2. The final Section endeavours to abstract from the previous material pointers to the control of thyroid cancer.

Routine Statistics

England and Wales

Figure 1 shows the age-specific mortality rates for thyroid cancer for males and for females for England and Wales in 1971–1975. With the mortality rate plotted on a log scale there is a near-linear increase with advancing age and a female excess over the male rates throughout the age range. This is one of the few cancers affecting both sexes in which there is an excess of female deaths. The data reflected in Fig. 2 are restricted to females, but this Figure contrasts the incidence with the mortality; at younger ages there is a considerably higher incidence rate, which gradually approximates to the mortality rate with advancing age. Figure 3 presents the trends in the age-specific rates for females in England and Wales for the period 1931–1975. Five age groups are plotted and there is a slight suggestion that the mortality has decreased for the middle three; these changes are negligible compared with trends for some other sites.

Campbell and Doll (1963) reviewed national data for England and Wales on incidence, survival, and mortality. They suggested that mortality was relatively low compared with incidence in persons under the age of 25, and that it increased until the age of 60, when the survival is about 50% in diagnosed cases. They pointed out that this difference could occur if the fatality of the disease was low in childhood and increased with age or if the ultimate fatality remained relatively constant, but the duration of survival was longer in younger patients. They also commented that clinical experience suggests that the prognosis varies greatly with histological type. These factors obviously influence the ease with which national statistics on the mortality from this condition can be interpreted.

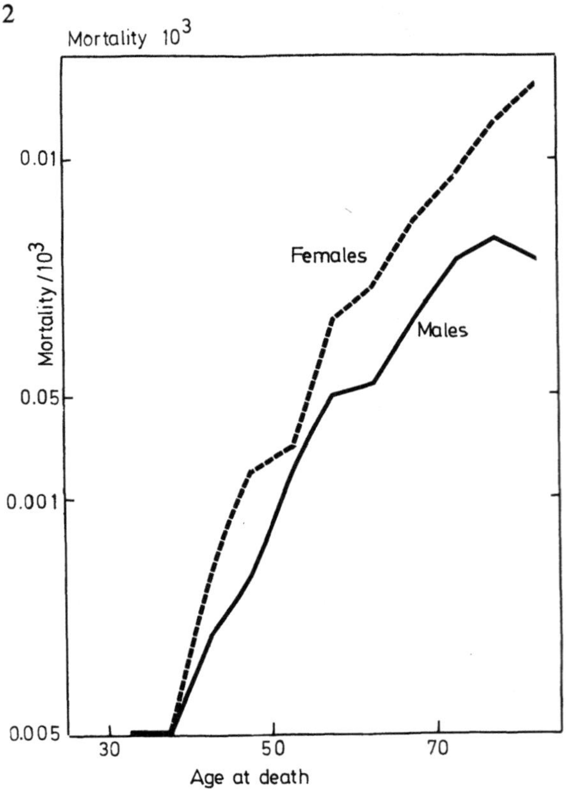

Fig. 1. Malignant neoplasm of thyroid: Mortality rates, 1971–1975, by sex and age at death, in England and Wales

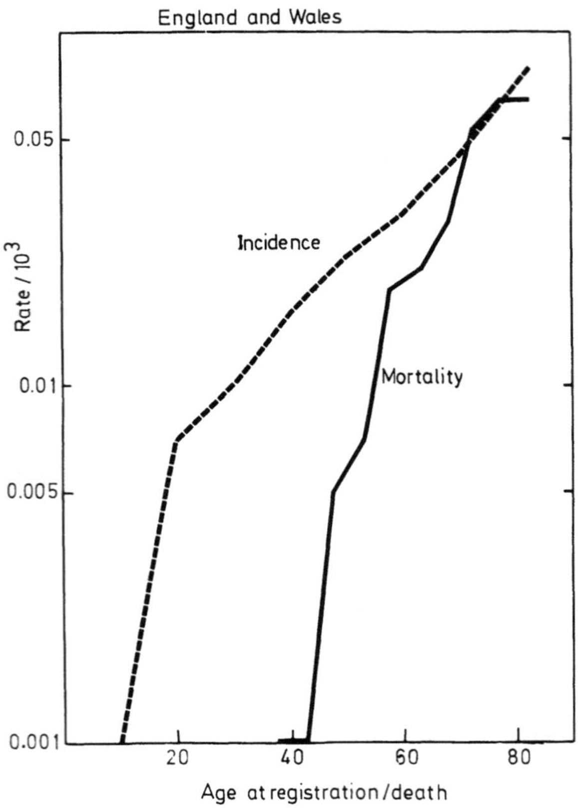

Fig. 2. Malignant neoplasm of thyroid: Female incidence (1970) and mortality (1973) rates by age at registration/death, in England and Wales

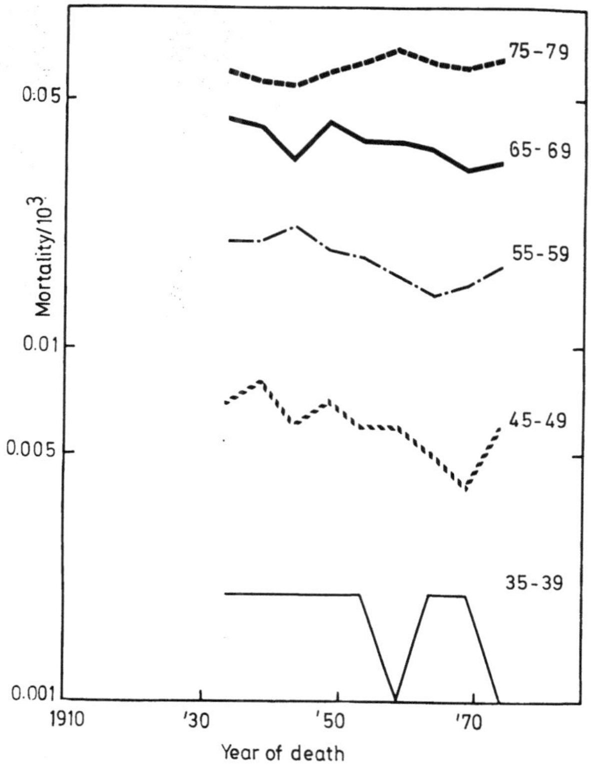

Fig. 3. Malignant neoplasm of thyroid: Female age-specific mortality rates by year of death, England and Wales, 1931–1975

Occupational Mortality

The Registrar-General's decennial supplement is published following the collection of data for each national census. Combination of the estimates of numbers of men in different jobs with an analysis of the causes of death for men by job permits the presentation of statistics indicating the association between occupation and mortality. There are a number of specific problems in the interpretation of this material, which have been discussed by ALDERSON (1972).

A general examination of the data, particularly for relatively rare conditions, is provided by a study of the social class distribution of mortality. Table 1 shows these data set out for males and females for the five standard social classes used by the Registrar-General; this table includes data from the 1931 decennial supplement onwards (Registrar-General 1938, 1958, 1971, 1978). There is no obvious social class gradient for either men or women, and the overall impression seems to be that neither at one point in time, nor over time has there been any appreciable association between social class and mortality from thyroid cancer.

Because of the relatively small numbers of deaths occurring annually in this country from thyroid disease, the detailed analysis of occupational mortality is of dubious value. For the 1959–1963 material there were only 250 deaths amongst men in the age range 15–64. Standardized mortality ratios (SMRs) were calculated for the 27 occupational orders, but obviously by the time the data are split between these there are relatively few deaths for any given occupational order – and yet the occupational orders are very broad categories of work and can imply considerable variation in environmental exposure from one group of workers to

Table 1. Standardized mortality ratios for thyroid cancer in males by social class in England and Wales. Registrar General 1938, 1958, 1971, 1978

	Social class				
	I	II	III	IV	V
1930–1932	125	100	106	100	86
1949–1953	100	119	98	97	88
1959–1963	88	112	100	80	138
1970–1972	157	106	92	113	109

another. In the published statistics (Registrar-General 1971) there is no occupation that is clearly identified as having a raised SMR; furnace, forge, foundry, and rolling mill workers have an SMR of 175, but this is based on seven deaths. Labourers not classified elsewhere have an SMR of 145, and this is based on 32 deaths. The latest analysis of occupational mortality (Registrar-General 1978) presented occupational units for which there was excess cancer mortality in 1970–1972 in England and Wales. Only one category, "Clerks and Cashiers", showed excess mortality for thyroid cancer; for men aged 15–64 the SMR was 168 and for those aged 65–74 the proportional mortality ratio (PMR) was 169. Because of the number of comparisons made (223 occupational units examined for each site), it is not clear whether this is a genuine reflection of risk of thyroid cancer in these workers or a statistical quirk.

International Statistics

Statistics on the incidence of thyroid cancer can be obtained from those population registries that cover localities or countries. In addition, some indication is given by special enquiries, which try to identify all known cases of a rare tumour. One of the problems with incidence data is that it is not known to what extent variation in reporting may be responsible for areal or secular variation in the statistics.

Another source of statistics is found in patients treated at a particular hospital. Miller et al. (1959) reviewed the increasing prevalence of thyroid cancer amongst their surgical patients and discussed the influence of institutional growth, institutional prestige, number of thyroidectomies performed, changing pathological criteria, improved clinical selection, and increased self-referral. It becomes very difficult to assess the influence of such factors, before commenting upon the trend in incidence in the population. Mustacchi and Cutler (1956) demonstrated how incidence might be estimated by aggregating data for hospitals and clinics serving ten metroplitan areas in the United States. They provided incidence rates broken down by race, sex, age, and region; limited analyses were also made by histological type. Renaud (1923) reviewed the cancer mortality statistics for Switzerland for the period 1901–1920. He did not present age-specific rates, but the proportion of cancer deaths due to neoplasms of the thyroid. This had fallen from 1.6% of all cancer deaths in males and females combined in 1901–1910 to 1.0% in 1911–1920. He suggested that this reduction might be due to earlier treatment of benign lesions of the thyroid in the latter period.

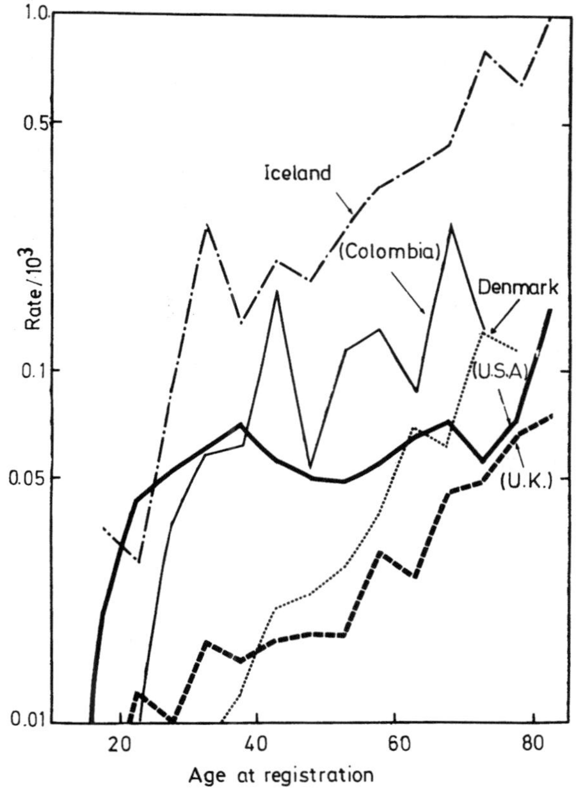

Fig. 4. Malignant neoplasm of thyroid: Female incidence rates, around 1970, by age at registration, in five countries. Where the country's name is in brackets this indicates the data are based on the incidence in selected regions rather than in the entire country

Using data from various publications, HAKAMA (1969) compared the incidence and mortality of thyroid cancer for a number of countries. The data were age-adjusted and were examined by sex. He commented that, with few exceptions, thyroid cancer showed a very similar occurrence all over the world. However, he concluded that very little could be said about the varying world incidence, because even the best sources of data indicate that the majority of the differences may be due to random variation, under which possible systematic effects are hidden.

DOLL (1969) examined the incidence of cancer in different populations for a whole series of sites; it is evident from a table in his paper that the range of incidence for thyroid cancer is relatively small compared with the variation that occurs for some other sites. Figure 4 is based on the statistics for five continents (WATERHOUSE et al. 1976); this shows about a tenfold variation in incidence, which is less than occurs for many other sites.

CARROLL et al. (1964) examined the incidence of thyroid cancer in New York State for the period 1941–1962; they showed that the rate had more than doubled in this period, but this had occurred only in persons under 55 years of age. For cohorts born after 1910 the rate at each age was approximately doubled for each successive decade of birth; there is then an indication that this increase has become less marked for the latest cohort for which they have data. They suggest, because of the nature of the changes, that an alteration of diagnostic acumen of diagnosis could not account for the increase and that some aetiological factor is more likely to be the reason. They suggest that the changes coincide with the use of X-ray therapy for thyroid enlargement in children (see section on therapeutic irradiation).

WINSHIP and ROSVOLL (1961) discussed the reported thyroid cancers in childhood; they identified patients both through the published literature and through personal surveys carried out in countries throughout the world. Altogether they reported 562 known childhood lesions, 315 from the literature and 247 obtained from special enquiry. Eighty percent of these children were resident in the United States, but there was no locality within that country where there was a particularly high incidence. SCHOTTENFELD and GERSHAM (1977a) disussed the incidence, survival, and mortality for the United States; they suggest that relative survival rates for both men and women improved substantially between 1940–1949 and 1960–1964. They infer from this that the age-adjusted mortality and the increasing age-adjusted incidence have declined because there have been more significant gains in survival and thus in the average duration of the disease.

Specific Problems in the Application of Routine Statistics on Thyroid Cancer

ALDERSON (1974, 1977) has reviewed the difficulties inherent in the use of routine mortality and morbidity statistics. Apart from the need to bear the general biases and errors of this material in mind, there are some specific problems with the data on thyroid cancer. Thyroid cancer is one of the conditions in which occult lesions can occur. SCHOTTENFELD and GERSHAM (1977a) discussed data derived from 5636 consecutive autopsies at the Memorial Hospital. Where no tumour was grossly visible the routine examination involved a single section from each lobe of the thyroid. An independent primary cancer was identified in 6.4 per 1000 autopsies, with a peak prevalence in women aged 20–29 (19.6 per 1000) and in men aged 30–39 (10.4 per 1000). The condition differs from most carcinomas, at they point out, in that there was no indication that subclinical thyroid cancer increases with increasing age.
In 3067 consecutive autopsies from the Hiroshima – Nagasaki lifespan study (SAMPSON et al. 1969), 536 primary thyroid carcinomas were found, 97% being occult papillary carcinomas. The prevalence was significantly higher in women and those exposed to doses of 50 rads or more direct atomic radiation, but it did not increase with age. The prevalence of occult thyroid carcinoma in 1096 persons with no recorded radiation exposure in 1945 was 17.9%, compared with the 1.0%–4.0% reported from various American series (Table 2). In view of this marked discrepancy, SAMPSON et al. (1974) studied the thyroids of 159 deceased residents of Minnesota, using the same techniques and pathology criteria; they found nine occult carcinomas of the thyroid, a prevalence of 5.7%. The authors did not think that differences in the sex ratio, the age distribution, or exposure to irradiation explained the findings. (There was an appreciable number of deaths in the Japanese series of subjects not known to have been exposed to the atomic bomb.) FUKUNAGA and LOCKETT (1971), in a comparable study, found latent papillary carcinoma in 24% of consecutive autopsies of Japanese adults in Hawaii. In a more extensive survey, FUKUNAGA and YATANI (1975) obtained thyroids from a series of autopsies in Canada, Colombia, Japan, Hawaii (Japanese dying there), and Poland. They demonstrated considerable variation in the prevalence of occult papillary carcinoma, despite the use of a standard histological technique.
A rather different approach was used by BERG et al. (1971), who reviewed autopsy records for a large sample of patients dying in 1952–1964 of a variety of malignant diseases. Just over 3% of these patients had a latent cancer, prostate, thyroid, colon, and kidney being involved particularly often. Serial sections had not been obtained and the identification of 36 thyroid cancers in 5636 autopsies is presumably a major underestimate of the true prevalence of la-

Table 2. Prevalence of latent thyroid cancer detected at autopsy in different countries

Country	Reference	No. examined	% Prevalence
Canada	FUKUNAGA and YATANI, 1975	100	6.0
Colombia	FUKUNAGA and YATANI, 1975	607	5.6
Japan	SAMPSON et al., 1969	1096	17.9
	FUKUNAGA and YATANI, 1975	102	28.4
Japanese in	FUKUNAGA and LOCKETT, 1971	100	24.0
Hawaii	FUKUNAGA and YATANI, 1975	148	24.3
Poland	FUKUNAGA and YATANI, 1975	110	9.1
U.S.A.	SAMPSON et al., 1974	159	5.7

Table 3. Prevalence of goitre and thyroid cancer in 59106 subjects in a non-goitre-endemic region of Japan, 1965–1970. After MARUCHI et al., 1971

	Prevalence/1000 subjects	
	Goitre	Thyroid cancer
Males	14	0.6
Females	54	1.9

tent cancers. Another approach was used by MARUCHI et al. (1971), who examined a large population sample in a non-goitre-endemic region in Japan. Nearly 60000 people were examined in 1965–1970 (this was over 80% of the selected population); all those who had a clinical abnormality were investigated further. Table 3 shows the prevalence of goitre and thyroid cancer found in either sex.

A quite separate issue is the influence of histology upon the natural history of thyroid cancer and the possible relationship between a specific aetiological agent and the development of a malignancy of a particular histological type. This is important for malignancies of many sites, but is difficult to explore on the basis of routine national or regional statistics, as the quality of the histological data is inadequate. This was clearly demonstrated by SAXEN et al. (1969), who re-examined and reclassified all thyroid cancer cases registered in Finland in 1958–1962. Of 392 patients, histology had been obtained initially for 89% – but for this study suitable material was only available for 92% of those whose condition was histologically confirmed (the biopsy was too small or "lost" for the remaining 8%). In only 122 of 345 (37.4%) was the same histological diagnosis confirmed.

They concluded that it was almost impossible to compare the incidence of different types of thyroid cancer in different regions unless the same pathologist had studied all the slides. In addition, they suggested that the frequency of papillary tumours is influenced by the activity of surgeons and cancer surveys, whilst the higher incidence of follicular carcinomas in endemic goitre regions is mainly due to overdiagnosis. CUELLO et al. (1969) showed considerable differences in the incidence of specific histological types when material from thyroid cancers in Cali, Colombia, and Connecticut, USA was reviewed.

Two what extent the improvement in diagnosis has been responsible for alterations in the national statistics is not clear. However, there is evidence that techniques for diagnosis, including interpretation of histology, have altered fairly radically during this century. The impact of these changes upon the statistics on incidence, hospital treatment, or mortality of thyroid cancer is difficult to determine. VERBY et al. (1969), in reviewing the trends in one United States county from 1935 to 1965, suggest that the rise in incidence can be accounted for by such "medical care" factors.

The Role of Genes

Race

Using national mortality and census statistics for the United States, FRAUMENI and MASON (1974) were able to examine the cancer mortality amongst Chinese Americans in 1950–1969. They showed an excess death rate from thyroid cancer, which was significant for males but not for females when compared with the death rates in whites und blacks (the risk ratios for males were 3.37 when compared with whites, and 4.16 against blacks, both with $P < 0.01$). However, the relatively limited variation in national statistics (compared with that for other sites) suggests that race is unlikely to be an important influence on risk of thyroid cancer.

Familial Studies

More specific examples of the genetic component in the aetiology of thyroid cancer come from two rather different clinical syndromes. The first is that of familial medullary carcinoma, a rare neoplasm that can occur as part of an inherited (autosomal dominant) syndrome with bilateral phaeochromocytoma (see HAZARD et al. 1959; BAYLIN et al. 1976; HILLYARD et al. 1978) Diagnosis of this neoplasm should be followed by screening of all living members of the family; this may be done by measuring the serum calcitonin level. A quite different constellation of abnormalities is found in the multiple endocrine adenoma syndrome; inheritance is attributed to a dominant autosomal gene. In an affected family members may suffer from adenomas and hyperfunction of the endocrine glands – especially the parathyroid, pancreas, and pituitary. SCHIMKE (1976) has provided a general review of these syndromes. JOHNSON et al. (1967) investigated a large kindred of 134 members in five generations; they identified only two thyroid tumours, and pointed out that the frequency of thyroid abnormalities in the general population made it difficult to assess the extra risk of thyroid disease in this syndrome. A specific association between thyroid carcinoma and phaeochromocytoma was first described by SIPPLE (1961). ALBORES-SAAVEDRA and DURAN (1968) described the association of thyroid carcinoma with chemodectoma. SCHOTTENFELD and GERSHMAN (1977b) have reviewed the importance of these genetically determined syndromes in the overall aetiology of thyroid cancer.

Amongst the 562 childhood cancers discussed by WINSHIP and ROSVOLL (1961) there were two families in which two members had been affected; in one family twin sisters and in the second family a brother and a sister had developed thyroid cancer. No indication is given as to whether this exceeds the expected frequency.

Association with other Diseases

SCHOTTENFELD and BERG (1971) investigated multiple primary cancers in a large series of patients from the Memorial Hospital, New York. On follow-up of 9792 women with breast cancer treated in 1949–1962, seven were found to have developed thyroid cancer; this was 4 times the expected incidence ($P < 0.01$). A smaller group of women with thyroid cancer subsequently showed a 50% excess of breast cancer, though this was not statistically significant. ITOH and MARUCHI (1975) demonstrated that a significant excess of breast cancer (compared with expected figures) developed in patients with Hashimoto's thyroiditis, but not in patients with myxoedema, hyperthyroidism, or benign nodular goitre. HIRABAYASHE and LINDSAY (1965) reported a statistically significant association between papillary carcinoma of the thyroid and chronic thyroiditis – but they point out that the latter may be secondary to the presence of thyroid cancer. The specific association of Hashimoto's thyroiditis and lymphoma of the thyroid is beyond the scope of this Chapter. SCHOTTENFELD and GERSHAM (1977b), in reviewing this and other reports, suggest the evidence is insufficient to confirm that breast and thyroid cancer have a common aetiology. Amongst the 562 children described by WINSHIP and ROSVOLL (1961) there were ten patients with reported coincidental disease (two were mentally retarded and harelip, congenital heart defect, poliomyelitis, asthma, brain tumour, lymphoma, and retinoblastoma were each found in one child). No expected figures are quoted and there does not appear to be any clear evidence from this of a syndrome of several associated diseases.

Thyroid Cancer and Goitre

WEGELIN (1928) pointed out that the percentage of autopsies that identified a thyroid carcinoma was related to the known prevalence of goitre in the locality (see Table 4). A number of studies have involved the parallel examination of national or regional data; CLEMENTS (1954) presented Australian data that showed no relationship between the mortality from thyroid cancer and either mortality from thyrotoxicosis or the incidence of goitre in the different states. SAXEN and SAXEN (1954) also found no association between the distribution of deaths from thyroid cancer and either the known prevalence of goitre or deaths from exophthalmic and toxic goitre. SMITHERS (1959), in reviewing published material, was satisfied that reduction of goitre by the introduction of iodized salt had lowered thyroid cancer mortality. PENDERGAST et al. (1961) found no association between the prevalence of goitre and thyroid cancer in the United States, whilst CORREA et al. (1969) noted major differences in these indices for a number of different countries. However, these last authors suggested that anaplastic carcinoma might predominate in areas with known endemic goitre. RAMALINGASWAMI (1969) discussed a number of problems associated with such studies and suggested that detailed analysis of the literature was futile.

A rather different approach is the histological examination of surgical and autopsy material. BEAHRS et al. (1951) presented the extensive data from the Mayo Clinic, gathered from over 13000 operations. Thyroid cancer was found in 0.5% of patients with exophthalmic goitre, 1.0% of patients with adenomatous goitre with hyperthyroidism, 4.8% of cases of nodular goitre, and 7.5% of patients with adenomatous goitre without hyperthyroidism. These authors do not discuss the interpretation of the varying prevalence of cancer. OLEN and KLINCK (1966) found cancer in 2.5% of over 2000 patients with thyrotoxicosis, which they say demonstrates a relationship – a rather extraordinary remark when they acknowledge that

Table 4. Proportion of autopsies revealing thyroid cancer, related to prevalence of goitre in different localities. After WEGELIN, 1928

Locality	% With thyroid cancer	Goitre
Berne	1.04	Highly endemic
Vienna	0.27	Mildly endemic
Prague	0.22	Mildly endemic
U.S.A.	0.11	Variable
Berlin	0.09	Rare

a higher prevalence of thyroid cancer has been reported from an unselected series of autopsies. WINSHIP (1967) suggested that foetal adenomas are the only lesions in the thyroid that can be regarded as precancerous. He indicated that they appear most frequently in women, predominantly in the age range 40–60, whilst they are extremely rare in children. In a relatively small series of 172 patients operated upon for Graves' disease, SHAPIRO et al. (1970) found 15 (9%) with previously unsuspected carcinoma; they suggest that the relationship between the two conditions may be underestimated in the literature, though their findings may be a reflection of chance variation.

The above two ways of exploring this topic can be profitably combined in studies of geographic pathology. WAHNER et al. (1966) examined the relationship of thyroid cancer to goitre in Cali, Colombia – where goitre is known to be endemic. They showed that the incidence (adjusted for age) was higher than in Puerto Rico or New York State, and that follicular and anaplastic carcinomas (but not papillary) were associated with nodular parenchymatous goitre. However, foci of carcinoma were found more frequently in extranodular tissue than within thyroid nodules. These data are compatible with a common aetiological agent, without the necessity of considering a sequential process from normality to benign thyroid disease, which subequently becomes malignant. WILLIAMS et al. (1977) have looked at the influence of high iodine intake, as there had been a suggestion that papillary cancer of the thyroid had been rising in Switzerland. They reviewed the histology of thyroid cancers in Iceland (a high-iodine-intake area) and Northeast Scotland (low iodine intake). The age-specific incidence rates for papillary cancer were 5 times higher in Iceland; there was a suggestion that follicular cancer was less common in Iceland.

Irradiation

Therapeutic

DUFFY and FITZGERALD (1950) reviewed 28 children with thyroid cancer. Only one came from a goitre-endemic area, whilst two had a family history of thyroid disease. Nine had had low-voltage X-ray therapy for an "enlarged thymus" between the ages of 4 and 18 months. In view of the number who had had such treatment, the authors state that this issue requires further study, though a cause-and-effect relationship cannot be proposed on this evidence. This initial (cautious) report was followed by a number of similar case reports from different parts of the world. GOOLDEN (1957) considered that it had by then been clearly established that irradiation of the thyroid in childhood increased the risk of subsequent cancer. CLARK (1955) reported 13 children with thyroid cancer, all of whom had had previous irradiation; RABINOWITZ and KATZ (1958) described a 12-year-old girl with cancer 7 years after repeated irradiation for "lymphoma in the neck"; WILSON et al. (1958) reported six patients with carcinoma of the thyroid following irradiation in childhood; in the same period (1946–1957) they had only treated a further six patients in the same age range up to 35. They also reported the occurrence of cancer in a woman aged 63, who had been irradiated for thyrotoxicosis when she was 26. Other reports were published by WILSON and ASPER (1960), WILSON et al. (1970), HARNESS et al. (1971), DEGROOT and PALOYAN (1973), BECKER et al. (1975). FRIEDLANDER (1907) first reported the use of irradiation for an enlarged thymus; during ensuing years an increasing number of children were so treated, and X-ray therapy was extended to other benign conditions about the neck. The puzzle is why the first report of thyroid cancer was only published in 1950, when the latent interval was often under 10 years. It is also a little difficult to see why these case reports continued to be published, when a major series of papers by WINSHIP and his colleagues had provided as much hard data from this approach as could be obtained. In their fifth publication on this work, WINSHIP and ROSVOLL (1961) reported an extensive postal survery of all children's and major hospitals in the United States and Canada and selected contacts throughout the world (in Western Europe, the Middle East, the Far East, and Central America). They hoped to identify all childhood cases of thyroid cancer. They recorded 315 published and a further 247 unpublished cases of thyroid cancer; only limited data were available for many, and a full history had been obtained for only 277. Of these, 221 had received prior irradiation for an enlarged thymus, hypertrophied tonsils and adenoids, haemangiomas, naevi, acne, eczema, cervical adenitis, and a number of other conditions. They noted that markedly fewer of the European children had received thymus irradiation.

Prospective Studies

A major improvement in estimation of risk stems from studies that have followed individuals given a known dose of X-rays. In a series of papers, HEMPELMAN et al. (1967, 1975) reported on the development of thyroid cancer amongst 2872 persons who received X-ray treatment in infancy for thymic enlargement. They contrasted their experience with observations in 5005 untreated siblings used as controls, and carried out a careful follow-up of subjects and controls. This was initially mounted by means of a mailed questionnaire to follow up the individuals via their parents or by direct address; nonresponders were telephoned. By 1971, responses had been obtained from 85.4%. Analysis of the earlier survey material had identified a specific group of individuals at high risk, and these have been followed by periodic survey to check for the development of thyroid cancer. PINCUS et al. (1967) have pointed out the variation in detection rate with different methods of assessing development of disease. A linear dose-response curve was apparent for the thyroid cancers, and it was shown that the incidence was much higher in those patients who had been treated with a combined anterior and posterior (AP) X-ray field. It was suggested that the AP treatment usually irradiated the gland with the primary X-ray beam, whilst in patients only having the A treatment the gland would only have been exposed to smaller doses of scattered X-rays. Excess risk of thyroid cancer occurred in female subjects, and especially in young adult females; there was no apparent age effect in the males. The magnitude of the thyroid dose could not be correlated with the latent period to tumour development; the 1967 report suggested a latent interval of some 20 years, by which time the incidence curve has risen sharply and then flattens off. However, the 1975 report suggests that the risk continued at least into early middle age. As part of this study, PINCUS et al. (1967) re-called a subgroup of the patients reported to have received a high dosage of X-rays for careful screening for any thyroid abnormality. They estimate that about one-third of 268 patients given a mean thyroid dose of 53 rads had developed thyroid nodularity. A number of other follow-up studies have been reported. SAENGER et al. (1960) identified children who had received irradiation for benign conditions in the head and neck region in four hospitals in Cincinnati in 1932–1950. Data were obtained for 1644 patients (73.7% follow-up) and 3777 sibling controls; thyroid cancer had developed in 11 of the patients (a 100-fold excess over the expected incidence) but in none of the controls. ALBERT and OMRAN (1968) followed up 85% of the children who had been treated by X-ray epilation for *Tinea capitis* in 1940–1959, and 79% of the control clinic population (well matched for age), who were treated by methods other than irradiation. They initially showed a higher incidence of head and neck tumours in the irradiated subjects; further follow-up until 1973 of 2215 treated subjects and 1395 controls revealed six thyroid adenomas in the irradiated subjects and none in the controls (SHORE et al. 1976). These authors' data suggested that the incidence was still rising with increasing length of follow-up. JANOWER and MIETIEN (1971) followed 466 children who had received irradiation to the thymus in the period 1922–1946, together with 506 unirradiated subjects with similar illnesses, and the sibs of both groups. Two of the irradiated subjects developed malignant lesions of the thyroid, no such lesions being found in the other subjects. REFETOFF et al. (1975) identified 100 patients who had had irradiation to the neck area (tonsils in 42%; adenoids 10%; tonsils and adenoids 7%; thymus 30%; acne 7%; other reasons 7%). There were palpable abnormalities in 26 patients; surgical exploration in 15 identified seven carcinomas. There was thus evidence that prior irradiation to the head and neck still constituted an important public health problem. In 1975, FAVUS et al. (1976) examined 1056 subjects who had been treated by therapeutic radiation for infection and inflammatory lesions of the upper respiratory tract in the 1940s and 1950s; the majority of these patients had received treatment to the tonsillar and nasopharyngeal region, and they represented 20% of the patients so treated. Nodular disease was detected clinically in 16.5% and by scan in a further 10.7%; 182 patients with nodular thyroids were explored surgically and cancer was detected in 60 of them.

MODAN et al. (1974, 1977) have reported on the development of thyroid cancer following scalp irradiation in about 11000 children who were treated for ringworm of the scalp in Israel. This group has now been followed up for a period of 12–23 years, and two categories of matched controls have been used – an equal number of nonirradiated subjects matched for sex, age, and ethnic background and a sample of nonirradiated matched siblings (approximately one sibling for every two cases). This work shows quite clearly that there is a relationship between radiation for scalp lesions and subsequent thyroid cancer, showing a linear dose relationship down to a level of at least 10 rads. MODAN et al. (1977) provided considerable detail on the estimation of dosage for individual children. They pointed out that though care has been taken to get the best possible estimate, special circumstances may have altered the specific dose exposure of the individuals who developed the thyroid cancer (e.g., fidgeting during treatment, variation in calibration, excessive irradiation time, or misplacement of shielding). WERNER et al. (1968) used a phantom to estimate the dose distribution following irradiation of the scalp. They suggested that the use of five fields at 350 R per field would give an average dose absorbed in the thyroid area of 6.5 rads. GESELL (1974) reanalyzed the data from Israel. He pointed out that the development of ten excess cases in a study population of 10902 subjects exposed to an average dose of 6.5 rads and followed for 23 years was equivalent to an absolute risk of 6.1 cases/10^6 man-rad years. This was important in demonstrating that the absolute risk rates calculated on higher doses also applied to these lower doses.

Administration to Adults

GOOLDEN (1958) reported two patients with thyroid cancer who had been given radiation in adult life (one woman treated at age 18 for thyrotoxicosis developed cancer when 36, and another treated when 28 for exophthalmic goitre was diagnosed as having a cancer 41 years later). This English report is difficult to assess, as thyroid cancer following irradiation in childhood had been much less frequently reported from England, but no data on numbers of exposed children or adults were provided. However, DELAWTER and WINSHIP (1963) traced 222 adults who had received thyroid irradiation for hyperthyroidism or other conditions. After follow-up averaging 22.5 years no evidence of any thyroid cancer was found; they suggested that there is a major difference in adults' resistance to radiation as a carcinogenic factor.

Control of Hazards

FUKS et al. (1976) have reviewed the effects of (therapeutic) radiation of the thyroid both from the aspect of induced thyroid dysfunction and from that of cancer development. They advocate periodic clinical and laboratory assessment of thyroid function and suggest that patients with elevated serum TSH levels should be given thyroid hormone to reduce hyperthyroidism and possibly lower the risk of thyroid carcinoma. The literature emphasizes that the predominant problem is in patients exposed as children. PIFER et al. (1963) estimated that about 18 of all babies born in the Rochester area in 1936–1945 were irradiated in infancy for an enlarged thymus. This poses a particular problem of contacting such at-risk subjects, as many will be unaware that they had this treatment. Despite the volume of publications, SOUTHWICK (1977) reviewed radiation-associated head and neck tumours and suggested that the full impact had been incompletely appreciated. FROHMAN (76) discussed suitable "control" of this long-term side effect and pointed out that lack of specific risk statistics and precise knowledge of the natural history of radiation-induced thyroid cancer had led to controversy over the steps to be taken. WALFSH and VOLPÉ (1978) suggest that about a quarter of all patients irradiated in infancy will have some thyroid abnormality, but they consider re-call of all exposed subjects impracticable, advocating in preference, "low-key education" of patients and consideration of potential hazards when these subjects are examined on follow-up. This is in line with the official policy published by the U.S. Department of Health, Education and Welfare (1977); the discussions of the workshop that led up to this have been summarized by the National Cancer Institute (1976).

Administration for Malignant Disease

In general, patients with malignant disease treated in the past with irradiation have been the subject of less concern, because of the prognosis of their primary cancer in relation to the risk of a second malignancy. There are a number of sites with good prognosis where this now becomes an important issue. SAGERMAN et al. (1969) followed up an appreciable sample of children treated for retinoblastoma. Six hundred and twenty-five patients were treated from 1930 to 1963; in general there was a policy of irradiation, according to a technique that has altered on two occasions. On follow-up they reported the development of thyroid cancer in two of these patients, and it is interesting to note that these two patients had a rather different treatment from the others; radium tubes on a tray were placed lateral to the eye for a predetermined period.

Radioiodine

A number of isolated case reports have been published of patients developing thyroid cancer following radioiodine (^{131}I) treatment for thyrotoxicosis (e.g., SHELINE et al. 1962; KARLAN et al. 1964; MCDOUGALL et al. 1971). These reports are difficult to evaluate, as the population at risk and the expected number of cancers are not known.

POCHIN (1960) has reported a follow-up study of some 60000 patients treated in the United Kingdom with radioiodine over a 20-year period. The emphasis of this follow-up was to identify the risk of leukaemia, but no evidence was found that leukaemia was caused by the radioiodine treatment. No reference is made in this work to the reported development of thyroid cancers. WERNER et al. (1961) published comparable data from the United States, with no indication of a thyroid cancer hazard. Between 1949 and 1967 about 35000 patients were notified to the English Cancer Registry as having received ^{131}I treatment for thyrotoxicosis. DONOVAN and ADELSTEIN (1974), in a brief abstract, state that after correction of errors in the data there was a slight excess in thyroid cancer mortality. No detailed analysis of this file of data has yet been published. STARR et al. (1964, 1969) followed 73 children and adolescents treated with ^{131}I; the majority were examined 10–18 years after initial treatment. One 12-year-old girl was found 2 years 4 months after her first dose of ^{131}I to have a papillary carcinoma, which was thought likely to have been present since before this treatment. HAYEK et al. (1970) reported the long-term follow-up of 30 children and adolescents treated between 1941 and 1968 for thyrotoxicosis with radioiodine. No deaths had occurred and there was no evidence of cancer or leukaemia in these patients. DOBYNS et al. (1974) reported on the Cooperative Thyrotoxicosis Therapy Follow-up Study, which involved patients treated between 1946 and 1964 in 25 centres in the United States and one in England, who were followed until 1968. Data were available for 98.8% of these patients, including primary treatment at the centres of 21714 with ^{131}I, 11732 by thyroidectomy, and 1238 by goitrogens for more than 1 year. As the study was only planned in 1961 there were some problems with interpretation, due to the local circumstances in referral of patients, selection of primary treatment in the centres, and follow-up investigations used to identify subsequent neoplasms. There were 59 malignant neoplasms found within 1 year of treatment; more than 1 year after treatment there were 19 amongst 21714 patients treated with ^{131}I, four amongst 11732 who had undergone thyroidectomy, and four amongst 1238 treated with antithyroid drugs. There is no significant excess risk in the ^{131}I-treated patients. There was no obvious relationship between age at treatment and risk of subsequent malignant neoplasm but a significant excess of adenomas occurred in those irradiated in the first two decades of life. SAFA et al. (1975) and SAFA and SCHUMACHER (1976) reported on the long-term follow-up (mean 11.3 years) of 108 children and adolescents treated with ^{131}I; they emphasize that there was no evidence of thyroid cancer and only one patient had developed a benign nodule. Recently, UTIGER (1978) has indicated that extensive studies have revealed no hazard of neoplasm from this therapy, but HOFFMAN and LUNDIN (1978) warn that this issue has still not been adequately studied, due to the possible long latent interval of radiation-induced thyroid cancer. JACOBSON et al. (1978) have assessed the contamination of the home environment by patients recently receiving ^{131}I therapy. They suggest that some children in the household might be exposed to a thyroid dose sufficient to double the risk of subsequent thyroid cancer.

MCKILLOP et al. (1978) have reported the development of a laryngeal cancer in a woman 8 years after treatment with ^{125}I for thyrotoxicosis. They were unaware of any case report of the development of a thyroid cancer, but indicate that this isotope might involve a greater risk of this hazard than ^{131}I.

Nuclear Warfare

HOLLINGSWORTH et al. (1963) described the thyroid abnormalities found in survivors of the Hiroshima atomic bomb during examination in 1958–1959 of 5553 adults. Twelve carcinomas were found in 168 subjects with abnormal thyroids (7%). Analysis of these limited data suggested that the patients were younger than usual; the eight female patients were under 50 and two of the male patients were 20 and 31 (the others being 64 and 65). There was a non-significant excess of patients in the high-exposure category. Following physical examination of the adult survivor population of Hiroshima and Nagasaki in 1958–1961, those with thyroid abnormalities were investigated further (SOCOLOW et al. 1963). Of 355 with enlarged glands, biopsy was initially advised in 141, but only 70 biopsies were performed (41 patients refused, 12 were not thought necessary by the surgeon, and 8 patients were "unavailable"). Twenty-one cancers of the thyroid were found, with a significant excess in those heavily exposed to ionizing radiation in 1945; 42% were in persons aged 30–39, though it was not clear whether this was due to earlier diagnosis or radiation induced acceleration of the pathological process. Further follow-up (WOOD et al. 1969; PARKER et al. 1974) confirmed the higher risk in women and those exposed in childhood, though the increased risk extended to those irradiated up to the age of 50.

JABLON et al. (1971) examined the cancer developing in children who had been exposed to the atomic bombs of Hiroshima or Nagasaki. In this study they had data on 15584 exposed survivors and 525 unexposed controls. Some data were available that made it possible to estimate the dosage received by the different categories of survivor, and there was a group of high-dose survivors (1109) who had received 100 rads or more. As indicated in Table 5, there was a significant excess of carcinoma of the thyroid in the exposed individuals, and a suggestion that this was associated with variation in the identified dosage.

In 1954, testing of thermonuclear devices in the Pacific resulted in exposure of the inhabitants of Rongelap Island to radioactive iodine in fallout; ^{131}I, ^{132}I, ^{133}I, and ^{135}I gained entry to the body by way of inhalation and food and water contamination (CONARD et al. 1966). It has been estimated that the adult thyroid dose was 160 rads from these sources plus 175 rads from X-radiation (with higher doses from iodine isotopes in children). At a survey in 1965, thyroid nodules were found in 11 of the people exposed to fallout in 1954, with no evidence of malignancy. On re-examination in 1969 (CONARD et al. 1970), in 67 exposed subjects 21 thyroid abnormalities had developed: three malignant lesions, 16 benign nodules, and two atrophic glands.

Table 5. Incidence of thyroid cancer by 1969 among 20517 survivors of children from Hiroshima and Nagasaki. After JABLON et al. 1971

Dose (rads)	Thyroid cancer		Relative risk[a]
	Observed	Expected	
0 –	5	9.9	1.0
10 –	5	2.9	3.0
100 + and unknown	5	2.2	4.5

[a] χ^2, 7.7; degrees of freedom, 2; $P < 0.05$

Diagnostic

BIRCH and BAKER (1960) reported a long-term follow-up study of 1480 children who had been exposed to repeat fluoroscopic examination in the course of care for rheumatic fever, congenital heart disease, or a few other unknown heart diseases. The average follow-up of all the subjects was nearly 18 years. Only two cancers were observed to develop during the follow-up period, which was below the expected incidence. There was no evidence from this study of an excess risk of thyroid tumours.

Occupational Mortality

Reference has already been made to the Registrar-General's occupational mortality tables. These provide no clear indication that people following any specific occupation are at high risk of developing thyroid cancer. INNES et al. (1969) reported that ethylene thiourea caused thyroid cancer in rats. SMITH (1976) carried out a study in the Birmingham region to check whether rubber workers, who are exposed to this chemical, were at high risk of thyroid cancer. A register of persons in the rubber industry was checked against the list of people in the Birmingham region who had developed thyroid cancer in the period 1957–1971. Though records were available for 1929 workers who had been at risk in the priod 1957–1971, no thyroid cancers were found in this group (though the expected number was not given in the report, it is very low). The only conclusion that can be drawn from this work is that there was no evidence to support a risk of thyroid cancer, though on the number of subjects involved the findings did not rule out a slight risk.

Conclusions

Bearing in mind the limitations of routine data on mortality and morbidity, which apply particularly to a condition like thyroid cancer, there is little evidence for changing frequency in England and Wales over recent years, and the international variation is relatively low compared with that of malignancy at some other sites. Some incidence data for New York State show an appreciable increase in cohort mortality for persons born after 1910.

A limited contribution to the overall morbidity from thyroid cancer comes from some specific genetic and familial syndromes, together with rare aggregations of several diseases including thyroid cancer. Earlier evidence that there was a relationship between endemic goitre and a high risk of thyroid cancer is not in accord with later data, and there is some indication of an excess of papillary carcinoma in localities with high iodine intake.

The main aetiological factor for which there is good evidence is X-irradiation of the head and neck. Long-term follow-up has shown that infants and children treated for a variety of conditions with X-ray irradiation, in particular, develop thyroid cancers (up to 100-fold the expected number). There appears to have been marked variation from country to country in the exposure of such patients, 1% of babies having been irradiated for thymus enlargement in some localities in America. There is no firm evidence of excess thyroid cancer in persons treated with ^{131}I for thyrotoxicosis, though no large-scale study with a sufficiently long follow-up has yet been reported for this hazard to be ruled out conclusively.

Present monitoring steps are restricted to screening members of families with medullary carcinoma and other genetic disorders, the regular surveillance of those exposed to X-rays – particularly in youth – and the avoidance of excess iodine intake. Current practice in therapeutic and diagnostic radiology results in restricted exposure compared with the past.

Despite identification of the above aetiological factors, the data available are not adequate to state confidently what proportion of all new thyroid cancers is due to each factor. However, it is suggested that the majority will be due to unknown causes. This poses a challenge to the epidemiologist, in conjunction with the pathologist and other scientists, to continue to explore this issue.

Acknowledgements. I am most grateful to Mrs. Christine Beaven for collating the routine data and preparing the artwork, and to Mrs. Pat Norton for the secretarial work involved. The Cancer Research Campaign's generous funding of the Division of Epidemiology made this work possible.

References

1 Albert RE, Omran AR (1968) Follow-up study of patients treated by X-ray epilation for tinea capitis. Arch Environ Health 17:899–918
2 Albores-Saavedra J, Duran ME (1968) Association of thyroid carcinoma and chemodectoma. Am J Surg 116:887–890
3 Alderson MR (1972) Some sources of error in British occupational mortality data. Br J Ind Med 29:245–254
4 Alderson MR (1974) Central government routine health statistics, vol II. In: Maunder WF (ed) Reviews of UK statistical sources. Heinemann, London
5 Alderson MR (1977) An introduction to epidemiology. MacMillan, London
6 Baylin SB, Gann DS, Hsu SH (1976) Clonal origin of inherited medullary thyroid carcinoma and phaeochromocytoma. Science 193:321–323
7 Beahrs OH, Pemberton J de J, Black BM (1951) Nodular goitre and malignant lesions of the thyroid gland. J Clin Metab 11:1157–1165
8 Becker FO, Economou SG, Southwick HW, Eisenstein R (1975) Adult thyroid cancer after head and neck irradiation in infancy and childhood. Ann Intern Med 83:347–351
9 Berg JW, Hajdu SI, Foote FW (1971) The prevalence of latent cancers in cancer patients. Arch Pathol 91:183–186

10 Birch AM, Baker DH (1960) Affect of repeated fluoroscopic examinations in 1480 children with long term follow-up study. N Engl J Med 262:1004–1008
11 Campbell H, Doll WRS (1963) The incidence of thyroid cancer in England and Wales. Br Med J 2:1370–1375
12 Carroll RE, Haddon W, Handy VH, Weiben EE (1964) Thyroid cancer: Cohort analysis of increasing incidence in New York State, 1941–1962. J Natl Cancer Inst 33:277–283
13 Clark DE (1955) Association of irradiation with cancer of the thyroid in children and adolescents. JAMA 159:1007–1009
14 Clements FW (1954) The relationship of thyrotoxicosis and carcinoma of the thyroid to endemic goitre. Med J Aust 2:894–897
15 Conard RA, Rall JE, Sutow WW (1966) Thyroid nodules as a late sequaelae of radioactive fallout. N Engl J Med 274:1391–1399
16 Conard RA, Dobyns BM, Sutow WW (1970) Thyroid neoplasia as late effect of exposure to radioactive iodine in fallout. JAMA 214:316–323
17 Correa P, Cuello C, Eisenberg H (1969) Epidemiology of different types of thyroid cancer. In: Hedinger CE (ed) Thyroid cancer. Heinemann, London, pp 81–93
18 Cuello C, Correa P, Eisenberg H (1969) Geographic pathology of thyroid carcinoma. Cancer 23:230–239
19 DeGroot L, Paloyan E (1973) Thyroid carcinoma and radiation. A Chicago endemic. JAMA 225:487–491
20 DeLawter DS, Winship T (1963) Follow-up study of adults treated with roentgen rays for thyroid disease. Cancer 16:1028–1031
21 Department of Health, Education and Welfare (1977) Irradiation related thyroid cancer: information for physicians. DHW Publication No. (NIH) 77–1120, Washington
22 Dobyns BM, Sheline GE, Workman JB, Tomkins EA, McConahey WM, Becker DV (1974) Malignant and benign neoplasms of the thyroid in patients treated for hyperthyroidism: A report of the co-operative thyrotoxicosis therapy follow-up study. J Clin Endocrinol Metab 38:976–998
23 Doll R (1969) The geographical distribution of cancer. Br J Cancer 23:1–8
24 Donovan JW, Adelstein AM (1974) Multiple-cause analysis of deaths of patients treated with radio-iodine. Br J Prev Soc Med 28:69
25 Duffy BJ, Fitzgerald PJ (1950) Cancer of the thyroid in children: A report of 28 cases. J Clin Endocrinol Metab 10:1296–1308
26 Favus MJ, Schneider AB, Stachura ME, Arnold JE, Ryo UY, Pinsky SM, Colman M, Arnold MJ, Frohman LA (1976) Thyroid cancer occurring as a late consequence of head and neck irradiation. N Engl J Med 294:1019–1025
27 Fraumeni JF, Mason TJ (1974) Cancer mortality among Chinese Americans. J Natl Cancer Inst 52:659–665
28 Friedlander A (1907) Status lymphaticus and enlargement of the thymus: with report of a case successfully treated by the X-ray. Arch Pediatr 24:490–501
29 Frohman LA (1976) Irradiation and thyroid carcinoma. Legacy and contraversy. J Chronic Dis 29:609–612
30 Fuks Z, Glatstein E, Marsa GW, Bagshaw MA, Kaplan HS (1976) Long-term effects of external radiation on the pituitary and thyroid glands. Cancer 37:1152–1161
31 Fukunaga FH, Lockett JL (1971) Thyroid carcinoma in the Japanese in Hawaii. Arch Pathol 92:6–13
32 Fukunaga FH, Yatani R (1975) Geographic pathology of occult thyroid carcinomas. Cancer 36:1095–1099
33 Gesell RF (1974) Radiation-Induced head and neck tumours. Lancet 1:815–816
34 Goolden AWG (1957) A review with special reference to radiation tumours in the pharynx, larynx, and thyroid. Br J Radiol 30:626–640

35 Goolden AWG (1958) Carcinoma of the thyroid following irradiation. Br Med J 2:954–955
36 Hakama M (1969) Different world thyroid cancer rates. In: Hedinger CE (ed) Thyroid cancer. Heinemann, London, pp 66–71
37 Harness JK, Thompson NW, Nishiyama RH (1971) Childhood thyroid carcinoma. Arch Surg 102:278–284
38 Hayek A, Chapman EM, Crawford JD (1970) Long-term results of treatment of thyrotoxicosis in children and adolescents with radioactive iodine. N Engl J Med 283:949–953
39 Hazard JB, Hawk WA, Crile G (1959) Medullary (Solid) carcinoma of the thyroid. A clinicopathologic entity. J Clin Endocrinol Metab 19:152–161
40 Hempelmann LH, Pifer JW, Burke GJ, Terry R, Ames WR (1967) Neoplasms in persons treated with X-rays in infancy for thymic enlargement. A report of the third follow-up survey. J Natl Cancer Inst 38:317–341
41 Hempelmann LH, Hall WJ, Philips M, Cooper RA, Ames WR (1975) Neoplasms in persons treated with X-rays in infancy: Fourth survey in 20 years. J Natl Cancer Inst 55:519–530
42 Hillyard CJ, Evans IMA, Hill PA (1978) Familial medullary thyroid carcinoma. Lancet 1:1009–1011
43 Hirabayashi RN, Lindsay S (1965) The relationship of thyroid carcinoma and chronic thyroiditis. Surg Gynecol Obstet 121:243–252
44 Hoffman DA, Lundin FE (1978) Does ^{131}I therapy for Graves' disease cause cancer? N Engl J Med 299:662
45 Hollingsworth DR, Hamilton HB, Tamagaki H, Beere GW (1963) Thyroid disease: a study in Hiroshima, Japan. Medicine (Baltimore) 42:47–71
46 Innes JRM, Ulland BM, Valerio MG, Petrucelli L, Fishbein L, Hart EH, Pallotta AJ, Bates RR, Falk HL, Gart JJ, Klein M, Mitchell I, Peters J (1969) Bioassay of pesticides and industrial chemicals for tumorigenicity in mice. J Natl Cancer Inst 42:1101–1114
47 Itoh K, Maruchi N (1975) Breast cancer in patients with Hashimoto's thyroiditis. Lancet 2:1119–1121
48 Jablon S, Tachikawa K, Belsky JL, Steer A (1971) Cancer in Japanese exposed as children to atomic bombs. Lancet 1:927–931
49 Jacobson P, Plato PA, Toereok D (1978) Contamination of the home environment by patients treated with iodine-131: Initial results. Am J Public Health 68:225–230
50 Janower ML, Mietien OS (1971) Neoplasms after childhood irradiation of the thymus gland. JAMA 215:753–756
51 Johnson GL, Summerskill WHJ, Anderson VE, Keating FR (1967) Clinical and genetic investigation of a large kindred with multiple endocrine adenomatosis. N Engl J Med 277:1379–1385
52 Karlan MS, Pollock WF, Snyder WH (1964) Carcinoma of the thyroid following treatment of hyperthyroidism with radioactive iodine. Calif Med 101:196–199
53 Maruchi N, Furihata R, Makiuchi M (1971) Population surveys on the prevalence of thyroid cancer in a non-endemic region, Nagano, Japan. Int J Cancer 7:575–583
54 McDougall IR, Kennedy JS, Thomson JA (1971) Thyroid carcinoma following iodine-131 therapy. Report of a case and review of the literature. J Clin Endocrinol Metab 33:287–292
55 McKillop JH, Doig JA, Kennedy JS, Thomson JA, Greig WR (1978) Laryngeal malignancy following iodine-125 therapy for thyrotoxicosis. Lancet 2:1177–1179
56 Miller JM, Horn RC, Block MA (1959) The increasing incidence of carcinoma of the thyroid in a surgical practice. JAMA 171:1176–1179
57 Modan B, Baidatz D, Mart H, Steinitz R, Levin SG (1974) Radiation induced head and neck tumours. Lancet 1:277–280

58 Modan B, Ron E, Werner A (1977) Thyroid cancer following scalp irradiation. Radiology 123:741–744
59 Mustacchi LP, Cutler SJ (1956) Some observations on the incidence of thyroid cancer in the United States. N Engl J Med 255:899–893
60 National Cancer Institute (1976) Information for physicians on irradiation-related thyroid cancer. C 26:150–159
61 Olen E, Klinck GH (1966) Hyperthyroidism and thyroid cancer. Arch Pathol 81:531–535
62 Parker LN, Belsky JL, Yamamoto T, Kawamoto S, Keehn RJ (1974) Thyroid carcinoma after exposure to atomic radiation. A continuing survey of a fixed population, Hiroshima and Nagasaki, 1958–1971. Ann Intern Med 80:600–604
63 Pendergast WJ, Milmore BK, Marcus SC (1961) Thyroid cancer and thyrotoxicosis in the U.S. Their relation to endemic goitre. J Chronic Dis 13:22–38
64 Pifer JW, Toyooka ET, Murray RW, Ames WR, Hempelmann LH (1963) Neoplasms in children treated with X-rays for thymic enlargement. 1 Neoplasms and Mortality. J Natl Cancer Inst 31:1333–1356
65 Pincus RA, Reichlin S, Hempelmann LH (1967) Thyroid abnormalities after radiation exposure in infancy. Ann Intern Med 66:1154–1164
66 Pochin EE (1960) Leukaemia following radio iodine treatment of thyrotoxicosis. Br Med J 2:1545–1550
67 Rabinowitz D, Katz J (1958) Carcinoma of the thyroid following irradiation of the neck. S Afr Med J 32:723–725
68 Ramalingaswami V (1969) Iodine and thyroid cancer in man. In: Hedinger CE (ed) Thyroid carcinoma. Heinemann, London, pp 111–123
69 Refetoff S, Harrison J, Karanfilski BT, Kaplan EL, deGroot LJ, Bekerman C (1975) Continuing occurrence of thyroid carcinoma after irradiation to the neck in infancy and childhood. N Engl J Med 292:171–175
70 Registrar General (1938) Registrar General's decennial supplement, England and Wales, 1931. Part IIa, Occupational mortality. HMSO, London
71 Registrar General (1958) Registrar General's decennial supplement, England and Wales, 1951. Occupational mortality. HMSO, London
72 Registrar General (1971) Registrar General's decennial supplement, England and Wales, 1961. Occupational mortality. HMSO, London
73 Registrar General (1978) Registrar General's decennial supplement, England and Wales, 1971. Occupational mortality. HMSO, London
74 Renaud A (1923) Quelques renseignements statistiques sur le cancer en Suisse de 1901 à 1920. Statistiques en general. Statistique Suisse. Rev Med Suisse Romande 43:433–450
75 Saenger EL, Silverman, Sterling TD, Turner ME (1960) Neoplasia following therapeutic irradiation for benign conditions in childhood. Radiology 74:889–904
76 Safa AM, Schumacher OP (1976) Follow-up of children treated with ^{131}I. N Engl J Med 294:54
77 Safa AM, Schumacher OP, Rodriguez-Antunez A (1975) Long-term follow-up results in children and adolescents treated with radioactive iodine for hyperthyroidism. N Engl J Med 292:167–171
78 Sagerman RH, Cassady JR, Tretter P, Ellsworth RM (1969) Radiation induced neoplasia following external beam therapy for children with retinoblastoma. AJR 105:529–535
79 Sampson RJ, Key CR, Buncher CR, Iijima S (1969) Thyroid carcinoma in Hiroshima and Nagasaki. JAMA 209:65–70
80 Sampson RJ, Wollner LB, Bahn RC, Kurland LT (1974) Occult thyroid carcinoma in Olmsted County Minnesota: Prevalence at autopsy compared with that in Hiroshima and Nagasaki, Japan. Cancer 34:2072–2076

81 Saxen EA, Saxen LO (1954) Mortality from thyroid disease in an endemic goitre area in Finland. Docum Med Geogr Trop 6:335–341

82 Saxen EA, Franssila K, Hakama M (1969) Effect of histological typing of registry material on the results of epidemiological comparisons in thyroid cancer. In: Hedinger CE (ed) Thyroid carcinoma. Heinemann, London, pp 98–103

83 Schimke RN (1976) Multiple endocrine adenomatosis syndrome. Adv Intern Med 21:249–265

84 Schottenfeld D, Berg JW (1971) Incidence of multiple primary cancers. IV. Cancers of the female breast and genital organs. J Natl Cancer Inst 46:161–170

85 Schottenfeld D, Gershman ST (1977a) Epidemiology of thyroid cancer, part 1. Clin Bull 7:47–54

86 Schottenfeld D, Gershman ST (1977b) Epidemiology of thyroid cancer, part 2. Clin Bull 7:98–104

87 Shapiro SJ, Friedman NB, Perzik SL, Catz B (1970) Incidence of thyroid disease in Grave's disease. Cancer 26:1261–1270

88 Sheline GE, Lindsay S, McCormack R, Galante M (1962) Thyroid nodules occurring late after treatment of thyrotoxicosis with radio-iodine. J Clin Endocrinol Metab 22:8–18

89 Shore RE, Albert RE, Pasternack BS (1976) Follow-up study of patients treated by X-ray epilation for tinea capitis. Arch Environ Health 31:21–28

90 Sipple JH (1961) The association of pheochromocytoma with carcinoma of the thyroid gland. Am J Med 31:163–166

91 Smith D (1976) Ethylene thiourea – a study of possible teratogenicity and thyroid carcinogenicity. J Soc Occup Med 26:92–94

92 Smithers DW (1959) Tumours of the thyroid gland in relation to some general concepts of neoplasia. J Fac Radiol (Lond) 10:3–16

93 Socolow EL, Hashizume A, Neriishi S, Niitani R (1963) Thyroid carcinoma in man after exposure to ionizing radiation. A summary of the findings in Hiroshima and Nagasaki. N Engl J Med 268:406–410

94 Southwick HW (1977) Radiation-associated head and neck tumours. Am J Surg 134:438–443

95 Starr P, Jaffe HL, Oettinger L (1964) Late results of I^{131} treatment of hyperthyroidism in 73 children and adolescents. J Nucl Med Allied Sci 5:81–89

96 Starr P, Jaffe HL, Oettinger L (1969) Later results of ^{131}I treatment of hyperthyroidism in 73 children and adolescents. J Nucl Med Allied Sci 10:586–590

97 Utiger RD (1978) Treatment of Grave's disease. N Engl J Med 298:681–682

98 Verby JD, Woolner LB, Nobrega FT, Kurland LT, McConahey WM (1969) Thyroid cancer in Olmsted County, 1935–1965. J Natl Cancer Inst 43:813–820

99 Wahner HW, Cuello C, Correa P, Uribe LF, Gaitan E (1966) Thyroid carcinoma in an endemic goitre area, Cali, Colombia. Am J Med 40:58–66

100 Walfsh PG, Volpe R (1978) Irradiation-related thyroid cancer. Ann Intern Med 88:261–262

101 Waterhouse J, Muir C, Correa P, Powell J (1976) Cancer incidence in five continents, vol III. International Agency for Research in Cancer, Lyon

102 Wegelin C (1928) Malignant disease of the thyroid gland and its relations to goitre in man and animals. Cancer Rev 3:297–313

103 Werner SC, Gittelsohn AM, Brill AB (1961) Leukaemia following radioiodine therapy of hyperthyroidism. JAMA 177:646–648

104 Werner A, Modan B, Davidoff D (1968) Doses to brain, skull and thyroid, following X-ray therapy for tinea capitis. Phys Med Biol 13:247–258

105 Williams ED, Doniach I, Bjarnason O, Michie W (1977) Thyroid cancer in an iodide rich area. Cancer 39:215–222

106 Wilson EH, Asper SP (1960) The role of X-ray therapy to the neck region in the production of thyroid cancer in young people. Arch Intern Med 105:244–251
107 Wilson GM, Kilpatrick R, Eckert H, Curran RC, Jepson RP, Blomfield GW, Miller H (1958) Thyroid neoplasms following irradiation. Br Med J 2:929–934
108 Wilson SM, Platz C, Block GM (1970) Thyroid carcinoma after irradiation. Characteristics and treatment. Arch Surg 100:330–337
109 Winship T (1967) Cancer of the thyroid gland. In: Raven RW, Roe FJC (eds) The prevention of cancer. Butterworths, London, pp 319–321
110 Winship T, Rosvoll RV (1961) Childhood thyroid carcinoma. Cancer 14:734–743
111 Wood JW, Tamagaki H, Neriishi S, Sato T, Sheldon WF, Archer PG, Hamilton HB, Johnson KG (1969) Thyroid carcinoma in atomic bomb survivors. Hiroshima and Nagasaki. Am J Epidemiol 89:4–13

Radiation Carcinogenesis

G. W. Dolphin

National Radiological Protection Board, Harwell, GB-Didcot, Oxfordshire, OX11 ORQ

Introduction

There are two important reasons for studying the risk of induction of thyroid cancer following irradiation. One is for radiological protection purposes, to help in setting radiation exposure limits for the thyroid in children and adults; the other reason is to assess the risk of thyroid cancer following radiation treatment of the head and neck region, which may include the thyroid in the primary or scattered beam, or the use of radioiodines in therapeutic or diagnostic procedures. The purpose of this paper is to review some of the existing data on radiation-induced thyroid cancers and to evaluate the risk.

Natural Incidence of Cancer

To assess the effects of radiation-induced thyroid cancer on a population, it is important to know the naturally occurring incidence and mortality in the population. The serial mortality tables by CASE et al. (1976) show that the mortality rate has hardly changed over the last 40 years in the United Kingdom. A summary of some data on the incidence of thyroid cancer in England and Wales, Japan, and Sweden, taken from the work of WATERHOUSE et al. (1976), is given in Table 1. These data show that thyroid cancer is a very rare disease in persons under the age of 30 years. The data on thyroid cancer incidence in England and Wales given by CAMPBELL et al. (1963) showed that the incidence was low compared with mortality in the younger age groups, but incidence tended to become nearly equal to mortality in older age groups. WINSHIP and ROSVOL (1961) studied 277 cases of childhood thyroid cancer and found that about 80% had a history of therapeutic irradiation.

Table 1. Annual incidence of thyroid cancer per million population. WATERHOUSE et al. 1976

Age group (years)	England & Wales		Japan		Sweden	
	Male	Female	Male	Female	Male	Female
10–15	0	2	0	0	0	6
30–35	3	3	0	23	10	26
50–55	8	24	9	55	24	55

Table 2. Histological types of thyroid cancer in an irradiated and a non-irradiated group ROUDEBUSCH and DEGROOT, 1977

Histological type	Irradiated (%)	Nonirradiated (%)
Mixed papillary follicular	64	60
Follicular	12	14
Papillary	20	25
Others	4	1
Number of patients	107	72

So far as radiological protection is concerned, the importance of this low incidence in the younger age groups lies in the inference that thyroid cancer caused by irradiation of children should be easily detectable against the background of the low natural incidence of the disease.

Histological Types and Prognosis

The spectrum of histological types of thyroid cancer is affected by the prevalence of goitre in the population, and an overall increase in cancer has been reported (DESMET 1960). ROUDEBUSH and DEGROOT (1977) have published some data on the histological types of cancer in an irradiated and a nonirradiated population, given in Table 2. There is a comparable spectrum for irradiated and nonirradiated persons, but there were no cases of undifferentiated cell cancers, and hence these data do not provide evidence on whether this aggressive type of cancer is induced by radiation more or less frequently than cancers of the differentiated type.

The prognosis following treatment for thyroid cancer is very good for the well-differentiated types, but HALNAN (1966) showed that the survival time tends to decrease with age at diagnosis of the cancer. Treatment of undifferentiated cancers is not very successful, particularly in older age groups, and the survival time may be only a few years. The survival following treatment is an important consideration, for the risk estimates used in radiological protection apply to mortality and not to incidence.

Latent Period Distribution

PARKER et al. (1974) have studied the incidence of thyroid cancer in the Japanese atomic bomb survivors surveyed in the Adult Health Study (AHS). People in this study are clinically examined biannually, and 40 thyroid cancers have been identified in the group of about 20000 people originally in the study. The distribution of the time of diagnosis for these 40 thyroid cancers is given in Table 3. The population is divided into those under 20 years of age at the time of the bomb (ATB) and those over 20 years. There is an indication that in the younger age

Table 3. Thyroid cancers and latent period distribution in the AHS (1958–1971)

Age ATP (years)	Total cancers	Latent period year			PYR[a] × 10^3
		< 5	5–15	> 15	
< 20	17	1	9	7	51
> 20	23	2	13	8	92

[a] Person year at risk

group the incidence is not falling with time and in the older age group there is a slight decrease with time. However, the statistical significance of this observation is marginal. HEMPELMANN et al. (1975), in their 1971 survey of individuals treated with X-rays to the neck region, found that 14 cancers occurred within 20 years of the irradiation and 10 between 20 and 40 years after irradiation. However, when expressed as a rate, in terms of person year at risk, the thyroid cancer incidence still appears to increase with time. Consequently the latent period for thyroid cancer following irradiation in childhood may be very long, or indeed there may be an increased likelihood throughout life that any cancer that develops will involve the thyroid.

Several studies have confirmed that there appears to be no correlation between latent period and radiation dose.

Irradiated Populations and Risk Estimates

In this paper the risk coefficient, R, for a group of irradiated persons who have received an average thyroid dose, D, is calculated from the following equation: $\frac{O-E}{n} = R \times D$, where O is the observed number of cancers, and E is the expected number, calculated from appropriate control groups. In this absolute risk estimate it is assumed that there is a linear relationship between biological effect and radiation dose at levels below a few hundred rads.

Irradiation of Marshall Islanders by Fallout

Three of the islands in the Marshall Group (situated in the Pacific Ocean) were accidentally exposed to fallout from the first hydrogen bomb exploded by the United States in Bikini Atoll in 1954. The people living on these islands were exposed to external gamma radiation from the fallout on the ground (CONARD 1977). The doses were 175 rads at Rongelap, 69 at Ailingnae, and 14 at Utirik. Many radioisotopes of iodine were produced in the nuclear explosion; some of these were inhaled directly and some of the longer-lived isotopes entered the body through the drinking water and local vegetable supplies, and concentrated in the thyroid. The dose from radioiodine varied with the age of the person; younger people received higher doses than older people due to the low mass of the thyroid in the younger age groups.

Table 4. Thyroid cancers in the younger and older age groups of Marshall Islanders (1954—1976)[a]

Island	Age < 10 years				Age > 10 years			
	No. at risk	Ob-served	Ex-pected	Dose (rads)	No. at risk	Ob-served	Ex-pected	Dose (rads)
Rongelap	23	1	–	1010	45	3	–	379
Ailingnae	6	–		382	12	–		135
Utirik	58	1	–	83	99	2	–	30

[a] R = $134/10^6$/rad (all data)
The cancers have occurred throughout a wide range of thyroid doses, all in females

Table 5. Some details of the cancer cases in the Marshall Islanders

Sex	Age at exposure (years)	Latent period (years)	Dose (rads)	Type[a]
F	6	15	905	P
F	16	22	425	P
F	21	15	335	P
F	29	11	335	M
F	4	20	70	M
F	21	15	31	F
F	37	16	31	M

[a] P, papillary; F, follicular; M, mixed P and F

The thyroid cancer incidence on the three islands is given in Table 4 for the two age groups under 10 years and over 10 years of age ATB. The mean value of R for all the data is 134 per million per rad.

Details given in Table 5 show that all the cancers have occurred in females, and the spectrum of histological types from this small sample is about the same as that in Table 2. Slightly more females were exposed than males, but the data clearly indicate that the female thyroid gland is more sensitive to radiation than the male gland.

In these data there appears to be no correlation between dose and latent period, and there is no evidence for a higher sensitivity to radiation among younger persons.

Japanese Survivors in the Adult Health Study (AHS)

As mentioned previously, 40 thyroid cancers were diagnosed between 1958 and 1971 in 20000 persons in the AHS (Parker et al. 1974). Of these cancers, 31 occurred in about

Table 6. Estimated risk of thyroid cancer in four groups of irradiated persons

Irradiated group	Number η	Observed/ expected	Average dose (rads)	Risk coefficient (per 10^6/rad)
Marshall Islanders	243	7	213	134
Japanese AHS	~ 10 000	23	115	20
Neck irradiation	2 872	24	119	70
Tinea capitis	10 402	10	10	92

Table 7. Distribution of thyroid cancers between the cities studied and between the sexes[a]

	Hiroshima		Nagasaki	
	M	F	M	F
Man rads $\times$ 10^3	250	380	210	310
Thyroid cancers	5	17	2	7

[a] Note that females are apparently more susceptible than males, and neutrons (at Hiroshima) are apparently more effective than γ-rays

Table 8. Distribution of histological types of thyroid cancer by age ATB

Age (year ATB)	No of thyroid cancers	Types of cancer[a]		
		P	F	M
0– 9	7	5	2	
10–29	18	12	6	
30–49	12	7	3	2
50+	3	3		

[a] P, papillary; F, follicular; M, mixed P and F

10000 exposed persons. At autopsy 34 more cancers were diagnosed, but only one death in the 40 diagnosed cancers has occurred.

The risk coefficient of thyroid cancer in the AHS is given in Table 6 as 20 per million per rad, on the assumption that the neutrons that delivered about 25% of the dose in Hiroshima had a relative biological effectiveness (RBE) for thyroid cancer of unity. If it is assumed that all the differences in cancer rate between the two cities can be ascribed to the neutron irradiation, an RBE for neutrons of about 5 may be deduced. In turn this value of 5 reduces the risk estimate to 17 per million per rad for low-LET (linear energy transfer) radiation.

In Table 7 the population doses for males and females in the two cities and the number of cancers are given. It shows that females are more susceptible than males and illustrates that the cancer incidence at Hiroshima is higher than that at Nagasaki, probably due to the greater effectiveness of the neutron radiation. The distribution of the histological types of thyroid cancer by age ATB is shown in Table 8.

Neck Irradiation in Infancy

Most of the 2872 persons in a survey reported by HEMPELMANN et al. (1975) received radiation for enlarged thymus glands in early infancy, which resulted in an average dose to the thyroid of 119 rads. During the follow-up period, which extends to almost 40 years, 24 cancers have developed. The calculated value of R is 70 per million per rad as given in Table 9, and the relative risk in female patients is 2.3 times that in males. Only one death attributable to thyroid cancer has occurred in the 24 cancer patients. HEMPELMANN et al. (1975) identified one particular group of patients who had all been treated by the same radiologist, who used a large X-ray field that included the thyroid in the primary beam. Most of the patients were Jewish and appeared to be at greater relative risk than non-Jews, with Jewish females having a very high relative risk.

Radiation Treatment for Tinea Capitis

During the mass immigration to Israel from 1944 to 1960, about 17000 children were treated for ringworm of the scalp by means of 75 or 100 kV X-ray generators. Doses were in the range 350—400 rads to the scalp. Measurements in a life-like phantom of the head (Werner et al. 1968) have shown that the mean dose to the thyroid as a result of this treatment was in the range 5—17 rads (Table 10). Over 10000 children have been followed for between 12 and 23 years, and data have been obtained on two matched control groups; from these a value, for the expected number E, of thyroid cancers has been derived. The excess of 10 thyroid cancers in this group gives a value for R of 92 per million per rad (MODAN et al. 1977).

Table 9. Risk of thyroid cancer following irradiation in infancy

No. of persons	Thyroid cancer Observed/expected		Dose (rads)	Risk 10^6/rad
2872	24	—	119	70

Table 10. Risk of thyroid cancer following irradiation of the scalp

No. of persons	Thyroid cancer Observed/expected		Dose (rads)	Risk 10^6/rad
10402	12	2	10	92

Therapeutic and Diagnostic Procedures with Radioiodine

DOBYNS (1977) described the U.S. Public Health Survey Co-operative Study of 30343 patients who were treated for hyperthyroidism with thyroidectomy, radioiodine, or drugs. Unfortunately, the mean follow-up time in the group of patients treated with radioiodine is only 8 years. In this group, 19 thyroid cancers have occurred, in some cases more than 1 year after treatment, in 19186 patients. Four of these cancers were anaplastic and six deaths have occurred from thyroid cancer.

The U.S. Bureau of Radiological Health has undertaken a co-operative study with 15 medical centres on the follow-up of 6800 children who received diagnostic doses between 1946 and 1968. These doses could have given rise to radiation doses in the range 20—200 rads to the thyroid. This dose range is of considerable importance in radiological protection, but unfortunately this survey will be of limited value due to the selection of children for diagnostic procedures.

There are many reports of thyroid cancer following treatments with ^{131}I, and a summary of these was given by MCDOUGAL (1974). However, it is not possible to draw any quantitative conclusions from such data, which usually concern isolated cases.

Conclusions

The R values for the four major irradiated groups of people are summarized in Table 6. R varies from 20 to 134 per million per rad. The lowest risk coefficient comes from the Japanese data, where follow-up time is limited, 1958—1971, and further thyroid cancers will probably develop in the population, thus increasing the risk coefficient. The high value in the Marshall Islanders may be due to high and early ascertainment resulting from the intense medical care given by CONARD (1977) and his colleagues. No allowance has been made for the expected number of cancers, and if this were needed it would lower the estimated value of R.

Estimation of the risk of thyroid cancer following treatment for hyperthyroidism involves two major uncertainties. One is that the study group is selected because of some malfunction of the gland which requires investigation, and this may mean that this group is at a higher than average risk of developing thyroid cancer. The other uncertainty concerns the radiation doses from radioiodine (^{131}I) treatment, which are very high and frequently lie in the range 5000—10000 rads. At this dose level most of the thyroid cells would be incapable of cell division, which is essential for the production of cancer.

For radiological protection purposes a value for R of $100/10^6$/rad is used to represent cancer incidence and a value of $5/10^6$/rad for cancer mortality. The evidence so far available supports the view that in younger people treatment for cancer is highly successful and that mortality is low. There are very few data on survival rates following treatment for radiation-induced thyroid cancers in older people. DOLPHIN (1968) suggested that children were more sensitive to thyroid irradiation than adults; the evidence now is inconclusive. However, there is no doubt that females are 2—3 times more sensitive than males. If females are twice as sensitive as males, then if R is $100/10^6$/rad for a population of equal numbers of males and females, then R is $66/10^6$/rad for males and $133/10^6$/rad for females. It may be prudent to take this into account in some aspects of radiological protection. Looking to the future, when neutron therapy of the head and neck may be used on a large scale, allowance must be made for the greater effectiveness of neutrons in inducing thyroid cancer. Apart from the Marshallese there are no data from human populations on the differences in the effectiveness of low-dose radioiodine

(^{131}I) irradiation and high-dose external radiation. The Marshall Islands data are too sparse to draw anything but the broadest conclusions on risk.

References

1 Campbell H, Doll WRS, Letchner J (1963) The incidence of thyroid cancer in England and Wales. Thyroid cancer. Br Med J 2:1370–1373
2 Case RAM, Coghill C, Davies JM, Harley JL, Hytten CA, Pearson JH, Willard SR, Alderson MR (1976) Serial mortality tables. 1. Anaplastic diseases. Institute for Cancer Research, London
3 Conard RA (1977) Summary of thyroid findings in Marshallese 22 years after exposure to radioactive fallout. In: DeGroot LJ (ed) Radiation associated thyroid carcinoma. Grune & Stratton, New York, p 241
4 DeSmet MP (1960) Pathological anatomy of endemic goitre. In: Endemic Goitre. WHO, Geneva, p 315
5 Dobyns BM (1977) Radiation hazard – experience with therapeutic and diagnostic iodine-131. In: DeGroot LJ (ed) Radiation associated thyroid carcinoma. Grune & Stratton, New York, p 457
6 Dolphin GW (1968) The risk of thyroid cancers following irradiation. Health Phys 15:219
7 Halnan KE (1966) Influence of age and sex on incidence and prognosis of thyroid cancer. Cancer 19:11, 1534
8 Hempelmann LH, Hall WJ, Phillips M, Cooper RA, Ames WR (1975) Neoplasms in persons treated with X-rays in infancy: fourth survey in 20 years. J Natl Cancer Inst 55:519
9 McDougal IR (1974) Thyroid cancer after iodine-131 therapy. JAMA 227:438
10 Modan B, Ron E, Werner A (1977) Thyroid cancer following scalp irradiation. Radiology 123:741
11 Parker LN, Belsky JL, Yamamoto T, Kawamoto S, Keehn RJ (1974) Thyroid carcinoma diagnosed between 13 and 26 years after exposure to atomic radiation. Atomic bomb casualty commission, Hiroshima, Jpn. Technical Report No 5–73
12 Roudebush CP, DeGroot LJ (1977) The natural history of radiation associated thyroid cancer. In: DeGroot LJ (ed) Radiation associated thyroid carcinoma. Grune & Stratton, New York, p 97
13 Waterhouse J, Muir C, Correa P, Powell J (1976) Cancer incidence in five continents. Publ international agency for research on cancer, Lyon
14 Werner A, Modan B, Davidoff D (1968) Doses to brain, skull and thyroid following X-ray therapy for tinea captiis. Phys Med Biol 13:247
15 Winship T, Rosvol R (1961) Childhood thyroid carcinoma. Cancer 14:734

Dysplasia and Neoplasia

D. S. Munro

University of Sheffield and Royal Infirmary, GB-Sheffield, S. Yorks S5 7AU

Introduction

Although carcinoma of the thyroid is relatively rare, clinicians who deal with thyroid disorders must never neglect the possibility of thyroid malignancy, either as the primary cause of thyroid enlargement or in association with another thyroid disease. There is no common thyroid disorder that is immune from occasional coincidental carcinoma, although most cases of thyroid malignancy arise in otherwise normal glands. Thus, published work on the association of thyroid disorders includes papers on carcinoma in simple goitre, solitary adenoma, multiple nodular goitre, thyrotoxicosis, and Hashimoto's thyroiditis.

In none of these conditions is the association particularly frequent, and it is more common to suspect malignancy in these patients than to confirm it. As will be evident from other chapters in this volume, none of the modern diagnostic aids will give absolute guidance as to the presence or absence of a carcinoma, so that the ultimate decision concerning the need for obtaining histology of a thyroid has still to be made on clinical grounds. Whether practising as a specialist in malignant diseases or as a physician with an interest in endocrinology, it is necessary to have a wide grasp of the pathological basis for the investigation of thyroid diseases. Many important aspects, particularly of the modern diagnostic methods, are fully dealt with in later chapters and are, therefore, omitted here.

An important baseline from which to consider the prevalence of thyroid malignancy in any particular group was studied by Mortensen et al. (1955) when they examined 821 clinically normal thyroids obained at autopsy and found 17 histologically malignant lesions. They concluded that occult carcinoma occurred about as frequently in clinically normal glands as in those with nodules. A similar incidence was observed by Silverberg and Vidone (1966), who examined 300 glands at unselected autopsies. The most important message that emerges from such studies is that careful histological examination of the thyroid will reveal an incidence of thyroid carcinoma far in excess of its clinical prevalence. In many of the conditions to be discussed later the opportunity for such examination has arisen as a result of thyroidectomy undertaken for the disease originally diagnosed, and the discovery of occult (clinically insignificant) carcinoma may exaggerate the real clinical problem of malignancy associated with benign or nonneoplastic thyroid diseases.

Developmental Anomalies

The thyroid gland is formed in a diverticulum from the pharyngeal floor and descends into the neck in the midline. The path of descent is usually obliterated but may persist in adult life as the thyroglossal duct, in which malignant tumours can arise. The literature relating to lingual thyroid tumours and infralingual thyroglossal duct tumours has been effectively summarized by SMITHERS (1970b). It is clear that carcinoma arising either in a lingual thyroid or in thyroglossal duct remnants is rare, as the total number of cases recorded up to 1970 is only 49. The follow-up data were badly incomplete and could not be used to assess prognosis in an individual patient. Clinically, the commonest developmental anomaly is a thyroglossal cyst, and the histology is almost invariably benign.

Simple Goitre

In contrast to the rarity of developmental anomalies, the commonest single thyroid disease is simple, nontoxic goitre. The precise incidence in different populations is difficult to ascertain, as the most commonly used technique for surveying populations is still inspection and palpation, which clearly means there is a substantial variation between observers. The distinction between endemic and simple goitre is often difficult and often depends on an earlier designation of a particular region as being one in which endemic goitre occurs. Certainly, in some areas of severe iodine deficiency almost everyone is affected, yet a recent survey in Sheffield (where severe iodine deficiency does not occur) showed an incidence of 5% in adult females (KILPATRICK et al. 1963). Some enlargement of the thyroid is a common finding in normal girls as they pass through puberty, and, like other thyroid diseases, goitre remains commoner in females at all ages.

Against this background, it is understandable that there are wide discrepancies between different assessments of the frequency with which malignancy occurs in simple goitre. The most striking feature of publications is the swing in emphasis that has taken place over the past four decades. At one time simple goitre was regarded as a common precursor of thyroid carcinoma, and the older papers often suggest that in goitrous areas (frequently known to be iodine-deficient) the incidence of thyroid carcinoma was substantially higher than in nongoitrous areas. For example, WEGELIN (1928) reported that thyroid cancer occurred 10 times more frequently in postmortem examinations carried out in Berne, which was known to be a goitrous area, than in Berlin. Many years later, WYNDER (1952) suggested that thyroid carcinoma had declined in Switzerland as goitre prevalence diminished after the introduction of iodized table salt.

On balance, studies in the United States of America have not supported an association between the two conditions. Indeed, PRENDERGAST et al. (1961) could not establish any relationship between the incidence of thyroid carcinoma in goitrous and nongoitrous regions of the United States, and when these authors compared the prevalence of goitre and thyroid cancer during World Wars I and II, their statistics suggested that the introduction of iodized salt, although effective in reducing the prevalence of goitre in some regions, had not significantly reduced that of thyroid malignancy, which had apparently increased slightly. Just as this evidence against an association appeared, papers from Colombia in South America (WELSH and CORREA 1960; CORREA and CASTRO 1961) suggested, quite strongly, that patients suffering from endemic or nodular goitre within the Cali Valley region had a distinctly higher incidence of thyroid carcinoma of the follicular or anaplastic types. There was also an absolute increase in all types of malignancy, however, which raised the question of the presence of additional carcinogenic influences in the area studied.

Such findings led WILLIAMS et al. (1977) to compare thyroid cancer in an iodide-rich area with that in an area of normal iodide intake. These authors chose Iceland and Northeast Scotland, centred on Aberdeen, because each of these areas had a well-defined population served by a single pathological laboratory. The most striking finding was a major difference in the incidence of papillary carcinoma in surgical specimens, which increased with age in both areas but was 5 times higher in Iceland (the area of high iodide intake) than in Northeast Scotland. Follicular carcinoma was rare in both areas but this tumour was relatively less frequent in Iceland than in Aberdeen. It was concluded that the evidence was compatible with the view that papillary and follicular carcinomas were separately influenced by variations in iodide intake. Undifferentiated carcinoma was 3 times as common in Iceland as in Northeast Scotland.

Thyrotoxicosis

In striking contrast to the swing of opinion that has tended to diminish emphasis on the association between simple goitre and carcinoma, the position with thyrotoxicosis is quite the reverse. Approximately three decades ago the view was consistently expressed that carcinoma of the thyroid very rarely occurred in patients with thyrotoxicosis and, indeed, it was thought that thyrotoxicosis might actually confer a protective influence against the development of malignancy. However, this view was first seriously questioned by SOKAL (1954) on statistical grounds, and from then onwards an increasing number of papers reported significant incidences of malignant change in thyroid glands resected primarily for hyperthyroidism. For example, OLEN and KLINK (1966) reported an incidence of 2.5% carcinomas in a series of 2114 thyroid glands resected for primary hyperthyroidism. This is comparable to the incidence reported in carefully examined specimens of nontoxic thyroids (MORTENSEN et al. 1955). In thyrotoxicosis, the majority of carcinomas were unsuspected clinically and were microcarcinomas of the occult type. LIVADAS et al. (1976) have stressed the importance of identifying "cold" nodules within the thyroid gland of patients with thyrotoxicosis, as they found that one-fifth of cold nodules in such patients were due to coincidental carcinoma. Encapsulated small occult sclerosing carcinomas were first described by HAZARD et al. (1949), who noted them as an occasional finding in Graves' disease. They are also seen in nontoxic goitres. Experience in Sheffield over the past three decades has tended to support the view that there is an elevated incidence of carcinoma of the thyroid in patients with thyrotoxicosis. However, before discussing the evidence, it is important to stress that the setting of studies on carcinoma in thyrotoxicosis may well be critical. Sheffield has a radiotherapy centre for a very large population and, just as malignancy in goitre may be identified by clinical factors, patients may be referred with thyrotoxicosis because of special clinical features. None of the patients described in Sheffield was found to have features of extensive functioning metastases from highly differentiated thyroid carcinoma, which must be relatively rare. The first Sheffield report published in 1957 reviewed 100 cases of carcinoma of the thyroid (KILPATRICK et al. 1957), and seven of these had thyrotoxicosis. A later report (HANCOCK et al. 1977) identified ten cases of thyroid carcinoma amongst 549 patients subjected to partial thyroidectomy for thyrotoxicosis in a 12-year period between 1960 and 1972. During this period an additional 936 thyroidectomies had been performed for other reasons (including suspected carcinoma), and in this group carcinoma was diagnosed in 110 cases. Of the 110 cases, approximately three-quarters had been suspected on clinical grounds of being due to a malignant tumour, and of the ten patients with thyroid carcinoma and co-existing thyrotoxicosis, no fewer than six had clinical manifestations that led to a strong suspicion preoperatively that there might be an associated malignancy. In the remaining four the disease was occult and was revealed only by histology. One of the six patients in the second series (HANCOCK et al. 1977), in whom the diagnosis was strongly suspected on clinical grounds before surgery, had received irradiation to the posterior fossa of the skull in infancy for a suspected tumour and thyrotoxicosis had been present for approximately 8 years before the diagnosis of carcinoma of the thyroid was confirmed at operation. There was increasing swelling of the neck, which, by the time the patient presented at Outpatients, was associated with obvious extension to the cervical lymph nodes. A radioiosotope scan with ^{131}I showed that uptake in the thyroid was limited to only one area of the thyroid itself, although, unusually, there was also radioiodine uptake in the microfollicular carcinoma invading the cervical lymph nodes. After radical neck surgery, which established that besides the microfollicular tumour there was diffuse toxic hyperplasia in the rest of the thyroid, ablative doses of radioiodine were given and the patient remains well some 4 years after her definitive treatment. In contrast, the earlier series from Sheffield included a majority of patients in whom carcinoma of the thyroid was only discovered after surgery, having been unsuspected clinically. Seven percent of 100 consecutive patients with carcinoma of the thyroid had thyrotoxicosis. Tumours were either papillary or follicular in type, and in five cases radioiodine concentration could be demonstrated in tumour tissue. However, only in two was significant remission in tumour spread induced by radioiodine therapy. In our second series the apparent benefits from radical neck surgery were slightly better. Four of the six patients appeared to have remission induced by a combination of surgery and treatment with radioiodine with subsequent suppressive therapy with thyroxine. In the four patients in whom occult neplasm was unexpectedly discovered at thyroid surgery the course was apparently benign, and following suppressive thyroxine therapy none of them had had any recurrence in the period of follow-up (which only extended to a maximum of 2 years at the time of our report). It is of interest that in six of the ten patients in whom we had diagnosed thyroid carcinoma associated with thyrotoxicosis we obtained blood samples for assay of the long-acting thyroid stimulator (LATS) and long-acting thyroid stimulator protector (LATS-P). These samples were obtained retrospectively, so that it is difficult to interpret the results, which showed an unexpectedly low incidence of these thyroid-stimulating immunoglobulins; only one of the six patients actually had significant levels of LATS-P. This is certainly lower than one would expect to find in a random sample of six patients with thyrotoxicosis, but it is known that following successful treatment of overactivity there is a tendency for the LATS and LATS-P levels to fall with time. It has been known for some time (Major and Munro 1962) that LATS can cause histological changes indicating thyroid activation and increase the cell division rate, as measured by the uptake of tritiated thymidine by the nuclei of thyroid cells exposed to LATS. It has, therefore, been suspected that perhaps prolonged stimulation of the thyroid gland by thyroid-stimulating immunoglobulins might well be relevant to the development of thyroid carcinoma, but direct evidence of this, so far as LATS and LATS-P assays are concerned, is lacking. The immunological disturbances associated with carcinoma of the thyroid and evidence of association with thyroid-stimulating immunoglobulins, as measured by assays dependent on blocking the binding of labelled TSH to sites on thyroid membranes by these immunoglobulins, is discussed in another chapter.

It is also relevant to consider the possibility that antithyroid drugs may be carcinogenic. There are publications based on studies in experimental animals (usually in rats) that suggest that goitres induced by antithyroid drugs may develop into metastasizing tumours if treated with carcinogens or radioiodine (Doniach 1970). An essential feature of the successful induction of these experimental thyroid malignancies was the creation of conditions in which excess pituitary thyroid-stimulating hormone (TSH) was secreted.

Although there are a few reports (Payne et al. 1947) of carcinoma of the human thyroid associated with exposure to thiouracil, this cannot be common in view of the extensive use of drugs of this type for many years. It seems likely that there are considerable species differences.

Autoimmune Thyroiditis and Lymphoma

Extensive lymphocytic infiltration of the thyroid was first reported by HASHIMOTO (1912); but Hashimoto's disease is not the only autoimmune thyroid disease in which such infiltration occurs; it is, for example, an almost invariable feature of Graves' disease, in which, although usually less extensive, the lymphocytic and plasma cell infiltration may correspond exactly to Hashimoto's original description (GREENE 1950; LEVITT 1951; WHITSELL and BLACK 1949).

Thus, it is not surprising that lymphoma of the thyroid gland occurs (SMITHERS 1970a), and attempts have been made to define the incidence of lymphoma in Hashimoto's thyroiditis (WOOLNER et al. 1966), in which carcinoma is also encountered (WOOLNER et al. 1959). There are also reports of lymphoma in patients with hyperthyroidism (SHIMOAKA et al. 1976).

Metastatic Carcinoma

Detailed postmortem examination showed that 9.5% of 1980 patients dying of malignant tumours at other primary sites had metastases in the thyroid gland. The majority of metastases were not evident on clinical examination (SHIMOAKA et al. 1962), although occasionally metastatic carcinoma may masquerade as primary thyroid cancer (ELLIOT and FRANTZ 1960) and it has been suggested that metastases in the thyroid may provoke hyperthyroidism (EDMONDS and THOMPSON 1978; SUNG and CAVALIERI 1973; VALENTA et al. 1970).

Conclusions

It is clear from this survey that there is no simple way of defining the interrelationship between thyroid malignancy and the commoner thyroid diseases. Modern diagnostic techniques do not identify with certainty the presence of malignancy in states of disturbed thyroid function. They may, however, give some clues to malignant change.

The most reliable principles for detecting malignancy in the thyroid remain the criteria obtained by simple clinical examination of a thyroid enlargement and its associated lymph nodes.

References

1 Correa P, Castro S (1961) Survey of the pathology of thyroid glands from Cali, Colombia – a goiter area. Lab Invest 10:39

2 Doniach I (1970) Experimental thyroid tumours. In: Smithers DW (ed) Tumours of the thyroid gland. Livingstone, Edinburgh London, pp 73–99

3 Edmonds CJ, Thompson BD (1978) Hyperthyroidism induced by secondary carcinoma of the thyroid. Clin Endocrinol (Oxf) 8:411–417

4 Elliott RME, Frantz VK (1960) Metastatic carcinoma masquerading as primary thyroid cancer. Ann Surg 151:551–561

5 Greene R (1950) The significance of lymphadenoid changes in the thyroid gland. J Endocrinol 7:1

6 Hancock BW, Bing RF, Dirmikis SM, Munro DS, Neal FE (1977) Thyroid carcinoma and concurrent hyperthyroidism. Cancer 39:298–302

7 Hashimoto H (1912) Zur Kenntnis der Lymphomatosen-Veränderung der Schilddrüse (Stroma Lymphomatosa). Arch Klin Chir 97:219

8 Hazard JB, Crile G Jr, Dempsey WS (1949) Non encapsulated sclerosing tumors of the thyroid. J Clin Endocrinol Metab 9:1216

9 Kilpatrick R, Blomfield GW, Neal FE, Wilson GM (1957) Carcinoma of the thyroid. Q J Med 102:209–233

10 Kilpatrick R, Milne JS, Rushbrooke M, Wilson ESB, Wilson GM (1963) A survey of thyroid enlargement in two general practices in Great Britain. Br Med J 1:29

11 Levitt T (1951) Evolution of the toxic thyroid gland. A clinical and pathological study based on 2114 thyroidectomies. Lancet 2:957

12 Livadas D, Psarras A, Koutras DA (1976) Malignant cold thyroid nodules in hyperthyroidism. Br J Surg 63:726–728

13 Major PW, Munro DS (1962) Observations on the stimulation of thyroid function in mice by the injection of serum from normal subjects and from patients with thyroid disorders. Clin Sci 23:464–475

14 Mortensen JD, Woolner LB, Bennett WA (1955) Gross and microscopic findings in clinically normal thyroid glands. J Clin Endocrinol Metab 15:1270

15 Olen E, Klinck GM (1966) Hyperthyroidism and thyroid cancer. Arch Pathol 81:531

16 Payne RL, Crane AR, Price JG (1947) Thiouracil and carcinoma of the thyroid. Surgery 22:496

17 Prendergast WJ, Milmore BK, Marcus SC (1961) Thyroid cancer and thyrotoxicosis in the United States. Their relationship to endemic goitre. J Chronic Dis 13:22

18 Shimoaka K, Sokal JF, Pickren JW (1962) Metastatic neoplasia in the thyroid gland. Cancer 15:557–565

19 Shimoaka K, van Merle AJ, Dindogin A (1976) Thyrotoxicosis secondary to involvement of the thyroid with malignant lymphoma. J Clin Endocrinol Metab 43:64–68

20 Silverberg SG, Vidone RA (1966) Carcinoma of the thyroid in surgical and postmortem material. Ann Surg 164:291

21 Smithers DW (1970a) Malignant lymphoma of the thyroid gland. In: Smithers DW (ed) Tumours of the thyroid gland. Livingstone, Edinburgh London, pp 141–154

22 Smithers DW (1970b) Carcinoma associated with thyroglossal duct anomalies. In: Smithers DW (ed) Tumours of the thyroid gland. Livingstone, Edinburgh London, pp 155–161

23 Sokal JE (1954) Incidence of malignancy in toxic and nontoxic nodular goiter. JAMA 154:1321

24 Sung LC, Cavalieri RR (1973) T_3 thyrotoxicosis due to metastatic thyroid carcinoma. J Clin Endocrinol Metab 36:215–217

25 Valenta L, Lemarrhand-Béraud T, Némec J, Griessen M, Bednar J (1970) Metastatic thyroid carcinoma provoking hyperthyroidism with elevated circulating thyroid stimulators. Am J Med 48:72–76

26 Wegelin C (1928) Malignant disease of the thyroid gland and its relations to goitre in man and animals. Cancer Rev 3:297

27 Welsh RA, Correa P (1960) The comparative pathology of goitre in a nonendemic and an endemic area. Arch Pathol 69:694

28 Whitsell FB Jr, Black BM (1949) A statistical study of the clinical significance of lymphocytic and fibrocytic replacements in the hyperplastic thyroid gland. J Clin Endocrinol Metab 9:1202

29 Williams ED, Doniach I, Bjarnason O, Michie W (1977) Thyroid cancer in an iodide rich area. Cancer 39:215–222

30 Woolner LB, McConahey WM, Beahrs OH (1959) Stroma lymphomatosa (Hashimoto's thyroiditis) and related thyroid disorders. J Clin Endocrinol Metab 19:53

31 Woolner LB, McConahey WM, Beahrs OH, Black BM (1966) Primary malignant lymphoma of the thyroid. Review of forty six cases. Am J Surg 111:102

32 Wynder EL (1952) Medical Progress: some practical aspects of cancer prevention. N Engl J Med 246:576

Control Mechanisms and Stimulation

C. J. Edmonds

University College Hospital and Clinical Research Centre, Northwick Park Hospital, GB-Middlesex, HA1 3UJ

Introduction

The introduction during recent years of radioimmunoassay methods has led to a considerable increase in our knowledge of the importance of thyroid and pituitary hormones in influencing the growth and function of thyroid tumours derived from the follicular cells. The present account is directed towards reviewing some of these advances, with particular reference to their clinical value.

The Normal Hypothalamic-Pituitary-Thyroid Axis

In the normal individual, control of thyroid growth and function is largely through a feedback system involving the hypothalamus and anterior pituitary. This has been extensively reviewed by several authors (e.g., Reichlin 1978) and will be only briefly considered here. A tri-amino acid peptide, thyrotropin-releasing hormone (TRH), is produced by the neurones of the medial-basal hypothalamus and secreted into the hypophysial-portal vessels. Thus TRH is carried to the anterior pituitary to control the formation release of thyrotropin (TSH) by the thyrotropic cells. Practically all phases of thyroidal iodine metabolism appear to be influenced by TSH, so that the uptake of iodine from the blood and the formation and secretion of thyroid hormones are all enhanced. There appears to be some thyroid function in the absence of TSH, but only at low activity (Ingbar 1972). The structure of the thyroid is also largely controlled by TSH, and the gland atrophies in its absence. The thyroid itself influences the TSH secretion rate through the feedback loop, the secreted thyroid hormones, L-thyroxine (T_4) and L-triiodothyronine (T_3), depressing TSH secretion, probably by actions both on TRH production and on the pituitary itself.

Iodine Uptake by Thyroid Cancers of Follicular-Cell Origin

Radioiodine has been used extensively in the treatment of thyroid cancers, because a high radiation dose can often be administered at little cost, both financially and to the patient's wellbeing. The efficacy of the treatment depends on adequate concentration and retention of the administered ^{131}I in the tumour itself. At first sight, this is unexpected, as thyroid cancers characteristically appear to be nonfunctioning when the patient is first seen, presenting, for example, as a thyroid mass that is "cold" on scanning. The explanation of the paradox lies in the effect of the removal or destruction of the normal thyroid gland. Almost invariably, the tumour function, as measured by its iodine uptake per gram of tissue, is very much lower than that of normal thyroid tissue at the blood TSH levels obtaining in normal people. Nevertheless, some degree of function is usual; fluorescent scanning, for example, generally demonstrates iodine in these tumours, albeit at low concentrations (PATTON et al. 1976). So that it is by comparison with the normal thyroid tissue that the tumour appears "inactive";

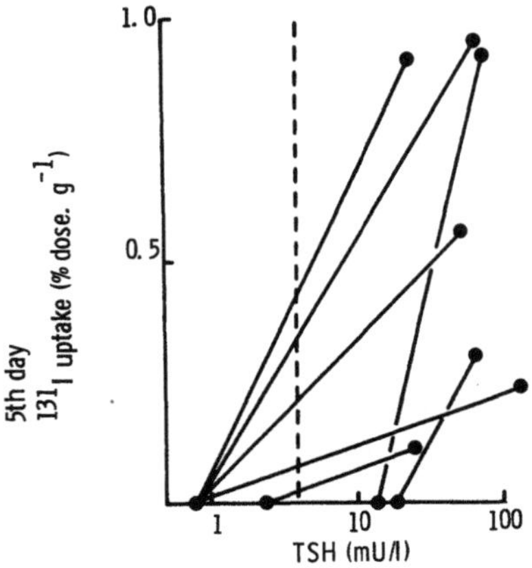

Fig. 1. Concentration of ^{131}I in differentiated thyroid carcinomas, measured in the primary site or in lymph node or bony metastasis before and after elevation of blood TSH level during induced mild hypothyroidism

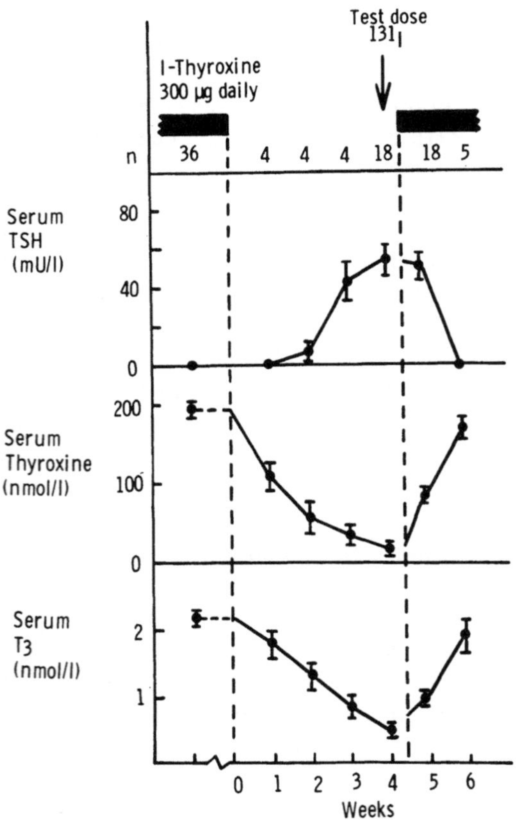

Fig. 2. Blood levels of TSH, T_4 and T_3 before, during, and after 4 weeks' withdrawal of L-thyroxine in athyreotic patients. *n* is the number of patients checked at each point. EDMONDS et al. 1977

once the normal tissue has been removed or destroyed, the functional capacity of the tumour becomes apparent. Furthermore, it can be clearly shown that tumour function very often rises considerably after ablation of the thyroid, and the factor of prime importance in producing this change is increased TSH stimulation (Fig. 1). The rise of blood TSH level results from the fall of the T_4 and T_3 concentrations in the blood following thyroid ablation or withdrawal of thyroxine replacement (Fig. 2). If TSH levels fail to rise adequately, something that does occasionally occur, as will be discussed later, tumour function generally remains poor. Since maximal tumour function is essential for effective ^{131}I therapy it is especially important to ensure that sufficient TSH stimulation is achieved when ^{131}I is given (EDMONDS et al. 1977). This is usually best achieved by withdrawing thyroxine for several weeks to produce mild hypothyroidism. Four weeks' withdrawal is adequate in most cases (Fig. 2), and involves relatively little discomfort as hypothyroid symptoms do not develop until the last week.

Suppression of TSH Secretion

As already indicated, TSH is important for the growth of the thyroid as well as for its function, and indeed probably plays a significant role in the development of simple goitres. Not surprisingly, therefore, TSH is also important as a growth factor for many thyroid cancers and it is a logical part of therapy to suppress this stimulant. Consequently, the usual practice is to give all such patients thyroxine in a sufficient quantity to suppress TSH production although, of course, without producing any hyperthyroid symptoms. This is ordinarily achieved with small doses, 200–400 μg L-thyroxine daily, little more than might be used for simple replacement treatment. Blood T_4 levels may then be near the top of the normal range, or even a little above, but blood T_3 levels remain within normal limits, the T_3 here being formed in peripheral tissues from deiodination of administered thyroxine. Doses have to be adjusted initially for individual patients, and we aim to give just enough to suppress the TSH rise that normally follows an injection of TRH, while ensuring that the serum T_3 level remains within the normal range (Table 1). This is possible in practice because a considerable degree of conversion of T_4 to T_3 appears to take place in the pituitary and hypothalamus, so that the TSH response to TRH is inhibited despite a normal blood T_3 concentration (WENZEL et al. 1975). If T_3 alone is used in suppression therapy, the interpretation of the hormonal levels is more difficult, because in the absence of any T_4, much of the T_3 is bound to the thyroid hormone-binding

Table 1. Thyroid hormone levels and TSH response to TRH 200 μg IV in 20 patients taking L-thyroxine

	Serum		TRH response	
	T_4	T_3	0 min	20 min
	(nmol/litre)		(TSH mU/litre)	
L-T_4 200–400 μg daily	164 ± 12 (SD)	1.8 ± 0.21	< 1	< 1
Normal range	60–150	1.2–2.8	< 1–4	8–30

serum proteins, leaving little of the important free T_3. Consequently, the blood T_3 concentration will appear to be well within the toxic range although the patient may both be clinically hypothyroid and have high circulating TSH values. Therefore, it seems that T_3 alone is less suitable for long-term maintenance, but if it is used careful supervision by means of TSH monitoring is essential (BUSNARDO et al. 1976). In our experience, the dose of thyroxine used in suppressive therapy for any individual patient appears to remain remarkably constant over years. We do carry out a yearly check of blood hormone levels, however, and this is particularly important during childhood and adolescence, when fluctuations are more likely and compliance may be slack.

Tumour Function and TSH Secretion

Some patients who have a relatively large mass of tumour, usually as metastases in lymph nodes in the neck or elsewhere, may develop considerable ^{131}I uptake associated with the development of a high concentration of protein-bound ^{131}I in the blood. This is of practical importance for two reasons. First, the liberation of a large amount of ^{131}I in hormonal and other organic compounds having a half-life of several days means the possibility of a large total-body irradiation dose. It may be necessary, therefore, to adjust the size of the administered therapy dose to eliminate this hazard. Secondly, it is generally found that despite the high uptake and protein-bound (PB) ^{131}I, the TSH levels remain high (Fig. 3). The explanation lies in the altered iodine metabolism in these functioning tumours. When stimulated by high levels of TSH they are capable of developing considerable iodine concentrations, but instead of this iodine being employed in the manufacture of thyroid hormones, it becomes attached to the plasma proteins, especially albumen, although the mechanism by which this occurs remains obscure (ROBBINS and WEATHERS 1966; POCHIN and THOMPSON 1969; TRIANTAPHYLLIDIS et al. 1969). The resultant iodinated protein has no hormonal activity and is therefore incapable of inhibiting the hypothalamic-pituitary thyrotropic axis (Fig. 4). The features are illustrated for one patient (Fig. 5) in whom the neck concentration of ^{131}I after thyroid ablation

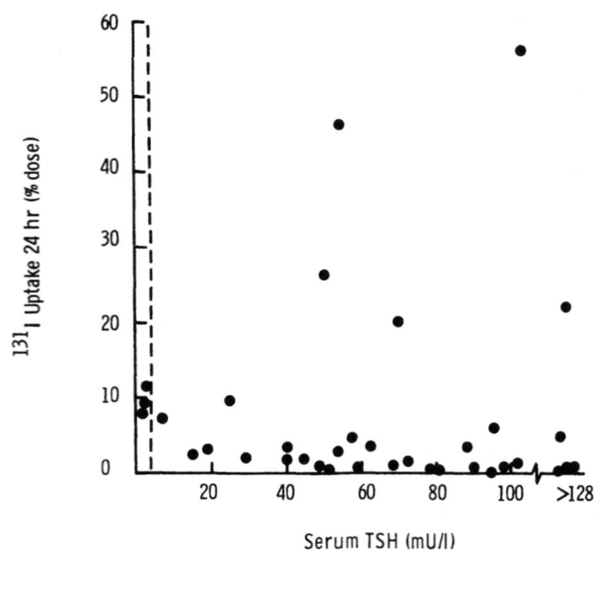

Fig. 3. Neck uptake of ^{131}I in relation to blood TSH level after surgery with or without ^{131}I ablation of any thyroid remnant. Note that some patients retain high neck ^{131}I uptake (concentrated in tumour) at this stage without inhibition of TSH secretion. The *broken line* shows the upper limit of normal for TSH concentration

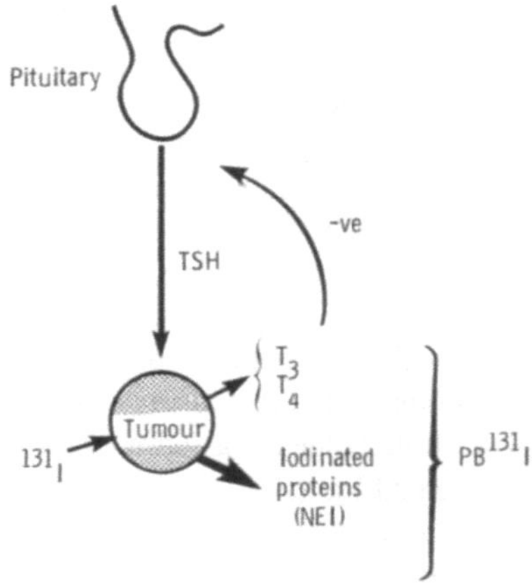

Fig. 4. Tumour stimulation and feedback (NEI, iodine compounds nonextractable in butanol)

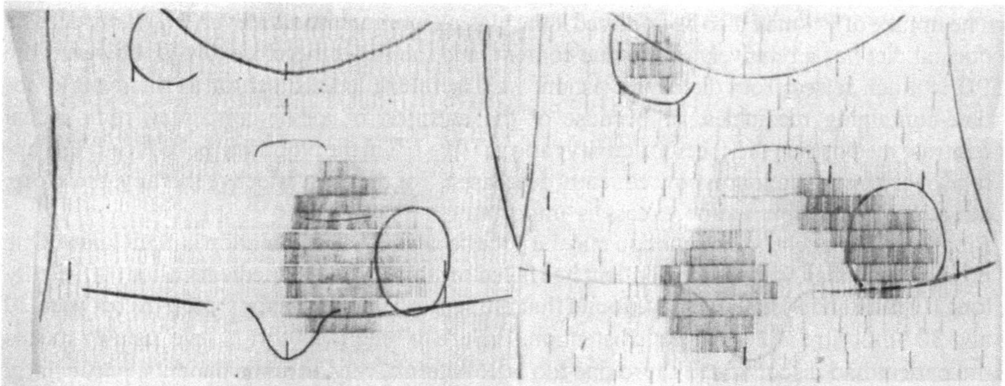

	12.02.74 Post lobectomy	02.04.74 Post ^{131}I ablation
Neck uptake (24hr)	42%	47%
Serum T_4 (nmol/l)	89	18
TSH (mU/l)	<1	54
PB^{131}I (%dose/l)	0.11	1.34
NEI	<0.01	0.69

Fig. 5. Illustration of events in a 22-year-old female patient. After initial lobectomy, uptake was localized in the normal remaining left lobe. After ablation of the latter with ^{131}I, neck uptake was the same overall, but localized in the tumour

was as great as before. Scanning showed, however, that the ^{131}I was now localized in the masses of involved lymph nodes. The thyroid hormone levels were very low despite the high ^{131}I uptake and the PB ^{131}I. Most of the PB ^{131}I was clearly not thyroid hormones, since a large proportion was insoluble in butanol.

Functional Characteristics of Clinical Importance

The radiation dose received by the tumour during ^{131}I therapy depends on the amount of radioiosotope taken up and the length of exposure to it. Thus the functional characteristics of practical importance are the ^{131}I uptake and its discharge rate from the tumour.

Experience has shown that the extent of uptake is related to histological appearances, although at present this relationship still remains rather crude. At one extreme there is the anaplastic cancer whose cells retain little if any iodine-concentrating property; at the other are the very well-differentiated thyroid cancers, which sometimes have an appearance closely resembling that of the normal thyroid and which concentrate iodine very well. In between, there is a whole range of variation of function in follicular and papillary cancers. In many of these, it is often difficult, initially, to be sure how much function will develop when hypothyroidism has been induced and blood TSH levels are high, but in a considerable proportion significant concentrating function is eventually demonstrable (Table 2). However, considerable histological and functional variation in the primary tumour and its metastases may be present; this is illustrated for one of our patients in Fig. 6.

The uptake of ^{131}I may also be impaired if the plasma inorganic iodide level (PII) is raised. The normal diet has a relatively low iodine content, and the PII is therefore low. If, however, the PII is much raised from dietary ingestion, e.g., by taking iodized salt or as the result of iodine-containing medicines, or because of the injection of iodine-containing radiological contrast media, then the specific activity ratio of $^{131}I : {}^{127}I$ in the blood will be reduced. The uptake of ^{131}I by the tumour is consequently decreased. For the most effective therapy, therefore, attention to possible iodine excess is important.

Finally, ^{131}I-concentrating function may be poor because TSH stimulation is inadequate. One possible explanation is that the patient has failed to stop thyroxine medication for sufficiently long. In most individuals we have found that the serum T_4 concentration drops to between 20 and 30 nmol/litre after 4 weeks' abstention. Failure to reach this sort of level usually means the patient had discontinued thyroxine too late. Alternatively, in some patients, particularly those who have been having thyroxine-suppressive therapy for some years, blood TSH fails to rise despite an adequate fall in the T_4 level (Fig. 7). The phenomenon is commoner in older patients and emphasizes the need to check thyroid hormone and TSH levels when test or therapy doses are given.

The rate at which the ^{131}I is discharged from the tumour is the other important functional variable. The turnover rate of ^{131}I has been observed to be considerably faster in thyroid tumours

Table 2. Development of ^{131}I concentration in tumour in 73 patients studied during the period 1970–1976

	Detectable initially	Detectable after thyroidectomy $\pm$ ^{131}I		
		Definite	Uncertain	Absent
No. of patients	6	29	28	10
% Dose per gram of tumour (estimated)	0.01–0.09	0.06–0.9	–	–
Blood TSH (mU/litre)	< 4	28–> 128	41–> 128	36–> 128

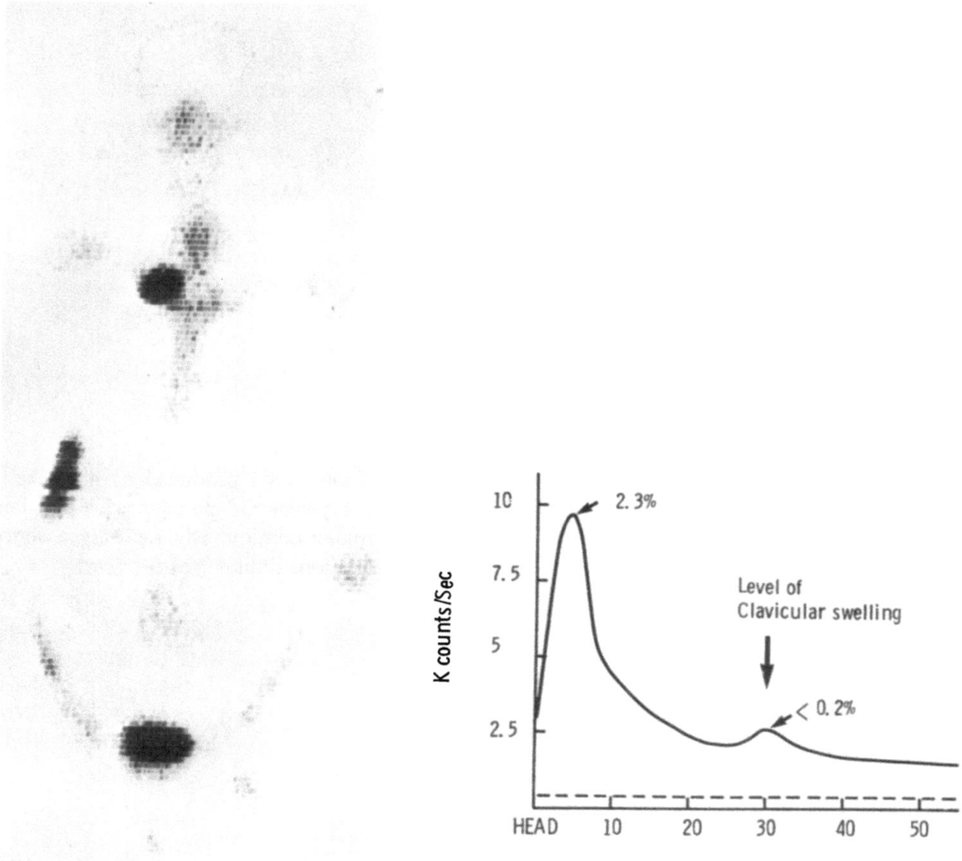

a b

Fig. 6. a Bone scan (^{99m}Tc pyrophosphate) of a woman with a follicular thyroid cancer treated 2 years earlier and reappearing with painful swelling of the sternal end of the right clavicle. **b** Profile scan after ^{131}I showed considerable uptake in an intracerebral metastasis (there were no definite neurological symptoms or signs) but very little in the clavicle

than in normal thyroid tissue (POCHIN 1971). This may be due to TSH levels being high at the time of study or to the differing metabolism of thyroid cancer cells. After a large dose of ^{131}I, the discharge rate is always relatively fast, the initial uptake halving in 3 days or less (Fig. 8). Radiation damage is probably an important causative factor in the accelerated discharge. This clearly places a serious limitation on the radiation dose that can be administered to the tumour.

Improving the Functional Characteristics

Improvement of the functional characteristics is of obvious value to ^{131}I therapy. Unfortunately, little can be done at present to improve the uptake by poorly differentiated tumours; the lack of differentiation is probably associated with the loss of significant biochemical

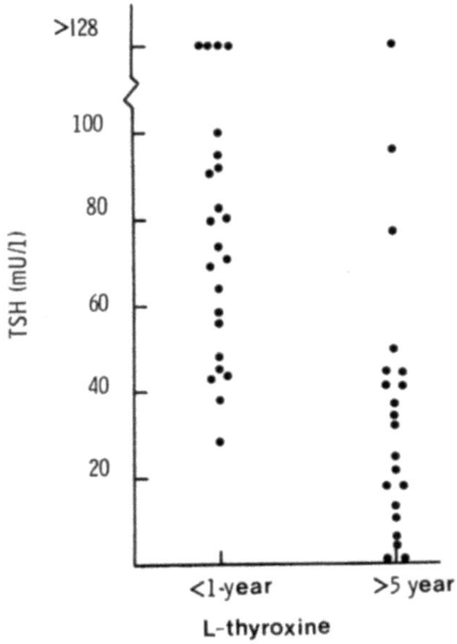

Fig. 7. Rise in blood TSH produced by 4 weeks' withdrawal of L-thyroxine in patients who had been receiving L-thyroxine continuously for only a short time (*left*) or for more than 5 years (*right*)

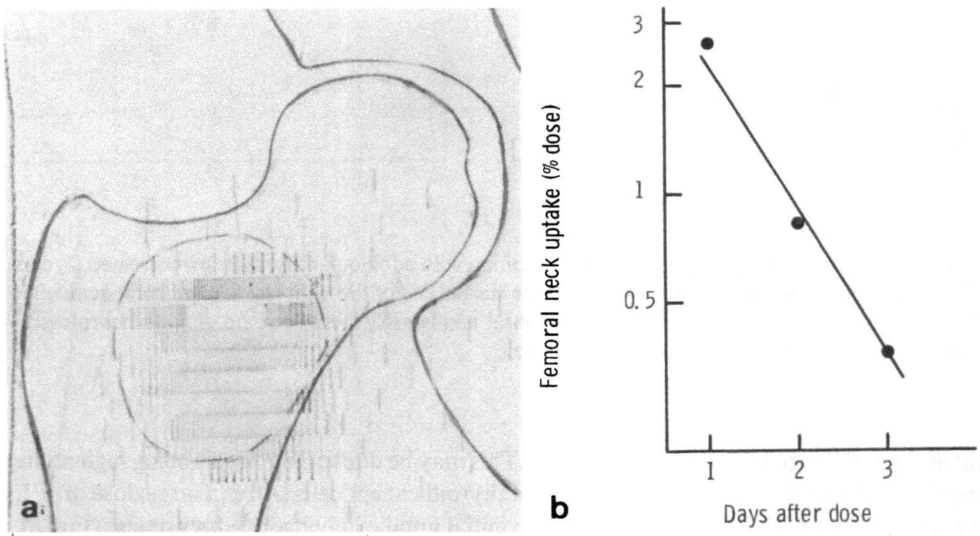

Fig. 8a, b. Fast discharge (**a**) of ^{131}I after a therapeutic dose (150 mCi) from a metastasis of follicular thyroid carcinoma present in the neck of the right femur (**b**)

pathways. But some well-differentiated papillary tumours also function poorly, and in them the explanation is less obvious. Deficiency of TSH receptors is one possibility, but the puzzle will remain unresolved until assays of the membrane receptors of tumour tissue are done.

It is important that the level of PII should be low. Preliminary diuretic treatment has been used in an attempt to increase iodide excretion and reduce PII (Hamburger and Desai 1966). The method has not been much used, but further investigations with newer diuretics seem worthwhile. It is important to ensure that ingestion of iodide is minimal, and patients are advised to avoid sea foods, iodized salt, and iodine-containing medication for 2–3 weeks before treatment.

The relationship between poor function and low TSH stimulation is especially important, since this is potentially remediable. Although the problem of restoring a patient's inadequate TSH response to thyroxine withdrawal has not yet been solved, the use of TSH given by IM injection for 3–5 days before ^{131}I is given will often produce a good uptake of ^{131}I (Hershman and Edwards 1972). There is some evidence for a negative feedback loop of T_4 on the thyroid (Yu et al. 1976), so that a period of preliminary withdrawal of thyroxine to reduce the blood T_4 level may improve the response to TSH. The routine use of TSH to stimulate ^{131}I uptake is a less desirable practice, as antibodies that can reduce its effectiveness form; occasionally, too, severe anaphylactic reactions occur. TRH has also been tried but has not proved sufficiently effective (Fairclough et al. 1973).

Lithium administration has been used in an attempt to reduce the discharge rate of ^{131}I while leaving uptake unaffected (Gershengorn et al. 1976). The method appeared effective when a small test dose of ^{131}I was used, but proved ineffective with large treatment doses. Unfortunately it is for the high therapeutic doses that the slowing of the discharge rate is needed. If the rapid discharge following treatment doses of ^{131}I is largely a consequence of radiation damage no easy solution is likely to be available. However, achieving a substantial reduction in the discharge rate would be so valuable for therapy that further studies of this aspect seem important.

Conclusions

Both function and growth of thyroid cancers originating from the follicular cells are, at least in part, dependent on stimulation by TSH. Although they usually function little at normal blood levels of TSH (< 4 mU/litre), when these are elevated following ablation of the normal thyroid and the induction of mild hypothyroidism, in many differentiated tumours function will be adequate for ^{131}I to be used in treatment. Daily L-thyroxine administration following thyroid ablation is used both as replacement therapy and also to suppress pituitary TSH secretion to prevent any stimulation of tumour growth. Withdrawal of L-thyroxine for at least 4 weeks is necessary to allow the blood thyroxine level to fall and TSH to rise to produce good tumour function. Some tumours develop considerable ^{131}I uptake and a high blood PB ^{131}I level, yet do not inhibit TSH secretion. This is because much of the concentrated iodine is abnormally handled by the tumour and relatively low amounts of active thyroid hormones are secreted. The ^{131}I uptake and discharge rate are important functional characteristics affecting the dose of radiation delivered to the tumour. Various factors, such as the degree of differentiation, the plasma inorganic iodide level, and TSH stimulation, determine these characteristics and they must be optimum when ^{131}I is used in treatment.

References

1 Busnardo B, Vangelista R, Girelli ME, Bui F, Lazzy C (1976) TSH levels and TSH response to TRH as a guide to the replacement treatment of patients with thyroid carcinoma. J Clin Endocrinol Metab 42:901–906

2 Edmonds CJ, Hayes S, Kermode JC, Thompson BD (1977) Measurement of serum TSH and thyroid hormones in the management of treatment of thyroid carcinoma with radioiodine. Br J Radiol 50:799–807

3 Fairclough PD, Cryer RJ, McAllister J, Hawkins L, Jones AE, McKendrick M, Hall R, Besser GM (1973) Serum TSH responses to intravenously and orally administered TRH in man after thyroidectomy for carcinoma of the thyroid. Clin Endocrinol (Oxf) 2:351–359

4 Gershengorn MC, Izumi M, Robbins J (1976) Use of lithium as an adjunct to radioiodine therapy of thyroid carcinoma. J Clin Endocrinol Metab 42:105–111

5 Hamburger J, Desai P (1966) Mannitol augmentation of ^{131}I uptake in the treatment of thyroid carcinoma. Metabolism 15:1055–1060

6 Hershman JM, Edwards CL (1972) Serum Thyotropin (TSH) levels after thyroid ablation compared with TSH levels after exogenous bovine TSH – complications for I-131 treatment of thyroid carcinoma. J Clin Endocrinol 34 (5):814–819

7 Ingbar SH (1972) Autoregulation of the thyroid: response to iodide excess and depletion. Mayo Clin Proc 47:814–819

8 Patton JA, Hollifield JW, Brill AB, Lee GS, Patton DD (1976) Differentiation between malignant and benign solitary thyroid nodules by fluorescent scanning. J Nucl Med Allied Sci 17:17–24

9 Pochin EE (1971) Radioiodine therapy of thyroid cancer. Semin Nucl Med 1:503–515

10 Pochin EE, Thompson B (1969) Metabolic activity of tumour tissue. In: Hedinger Chr (ed) Thyroid cancer. Springer, Berlin Heidelberg New York (UICC monograph, vol 12, pp 103–109)

11 Reichlin S (1978) Neuroendocrine control. In: Werner SC, Ingbar SH (eds) The thyroid. Harper & Row, Maryland New York London, pp 151–173

12 Robbins J, Weathers B (1966) Iodinated serum proteins in functional thyroid carcinoma. Cancer Research 26:570–577

13 Triantaphyllidis E, Thompson BD, Barnaby CF, Jasani B (1969) Iodination of serum proteins in vivo: relationship to irradiation and hypertrophy of the thyroid. J Endocrinol 44:467–474

14 Wenzel KW, Meinhold H, Schleusener H (1975) Different effects of oral doses of triiodothyronine or thyroxine on the inhibition of thyrotrophin releasing hormone (TRH) mediated thyrotrophin (TSH) response in man. Acta Endocrinol 80:42–48

15 Yu S, Friedman Y, Richman R, Burke G (1976) Altered thyroidal responsivity to thyrotropin induced by circulating thyroid hormones. J Clin Invest 57:745–755

Pathologic and Natural History

E. D. Williams

Welsh National School of Medicine and University Hospital of Wales,
GB-Cardiff, Wales CF4 4XW

Introduction

Cancer of the thyroid spans the whole spectrum of malignancy, some tumours being extremely slow-growing and compatible with an almost normal life expectancy despite the presence of metastasis, while other tumours show an extremely aggressive behaviour with death following diagnosis often in a matter of weeks or months. When it is considered, in addition, that malignant disease of the thyroid is derived from several different cell types it is obvious that any discussion of the natural history of thyroid cancer must be preceded by discussion of the pathological classification of thyroid malignancy.

Pathology

The major epithelial cell types in the thyroid are the follicular cell, derived from the thyroglossal duct and concerned with the production of thyroxine and tri-iodothyronine, and the parafollicular or C-cell, which is derived from the neural crest and is concerned with the production of calcitonin. The major controlling mechanisms of these two cell types are of course different, the first being responsive to TSH and the second to the level of serum calcium. It is important, therefore, in discussing the pathology of the thyroid, to separate the carcinomas into those of follicular-cell origin and those of C-cell origin. Follicular cells form the bulk of the cellular constituents of the thyroid, and follicular-cell malignancies account for 90% or more of thyroid carcinomas. C-cells are difficult to identify in man, and probably account for less than 1% of the epithelial constituents of the thyroid gland. C-cell tumours, however, form up to 10% of thyroid carcinomas. Tumours derived from both follicular and parafollicular cells may show varying degrees of differentiation. In C-cell malignancy (medullary carcinomas), the poorly and well-differentiated groups are not clearly demarcated, and although various histological features may be used to give an indication of prognosis the subgroups are not separately classifed. In contrast, tumours of follicular-cell origin show an unusually clear demarcation into the well-differentiated carcinomas with a good (often extremely good) prognosis and undifferentiated carcinomas with an extremely bad prognosis.
The differentiated carcinomas derived from the follicular cell are further subdivided into two broad groups on the basis of their biological behaviour. Papillary carcinomas are typically multifocal, not encapsulated, invading the lymphatics and metastasizing to local lymph nodes. Histologically they contain a papillary component, which may be dominant or minor. Follicular carcinoma is typically solitary and encapsulated; it invades veins and, when it metastasizes, often involves bones. Histology shows that it lacks a papillary component and is

composed in varying amounts of follicles and solid or trabecular areas. It is perhaps unfortunate that the terms papillary and follicular are used in this way, but this distinction is accepted by the WHO Classification (HEDINGER and SOBIN 1974); it might be possible to avoid confusion by remembering the two distinct uses of the terms papillary and follicular, as purely descriptive terms referring to the appropriate microscopic architecture and as diagnostic terms when they carry the connotation referred to above. If this distinction is remembered, such phrases as "a papillary carcinoma composed largely of follicles" may not appear confusing.

Undifferentiated carcinomas have also been subdivided on the basis of their microscopic appearance into spindle- and giant-cell carcinomas and small-cell carcinomas. It is becoming generally accepted that most small-cell carcinomas are malignant lymphomas, and it is apparent that some of the difficulty in diagnosis has been caused by the varied appearance resulting from the survival of partly or completely disrupted follicles. The typical anaplastic carcinoma shows an extremely pleomorphic spindle- and giant-cell appearance with numerous mitoses, an appearance in keeping with its highly malignant behaviour. In routine pathological studies of anaplastic carcinoma, evidence of pre-existing papillary or follicular carcinoma may be found in about one-third of cases. In studies where the whole gland was sectioned it was found that all the undifferentiated carcinomas examined in this way showed evidence of papillary or follicular carcinoma, which was interpreted as ante-dating the anaplastic carcinoma (IBANEZ et al. 1966). It seems likely therefore, as these authors suggested, that all cases of undifferentiated carcinomas of the thyroid arise from pre-existing differentiated carcinoma. Clearly this observation is of considerable importance in any discussion of the natural history of thyroid carcinoma. Except for malignant lymphoma, primary sarcomas of the thyroid are extremely rare. While there is some argument as to the most frequent type of malignant lymphoma found in the thyroid, it is generally accepted that Hodgkin's disease as a primary thyroid tumour is extremely rare. In some parts of the world malignant lymphomas may form up to 10% of all thyroid malignancies.

In much of the early work on the natural history of thyroid cancer the disease was discussed as if it were a single entity. It is clear from the foregoing discussion on pathology that the natural history and aetiology of each of the various types of thyroid cancer must be discussed separately. If they are fused and discussed as a single entity a great deal of information is likely to be lost.

Papillary Carcinoma

Papillary carcinoma makes up between 30% and 70% of thyroid carcinomas. In the large Mayo Clinic series (WOOLNER et al. 1961) it showed a very wide age range (5—85 years), with a mean age at presentation of 42 years. The sex ratio in this series was 2.4 : 1 (female : male). A number of factors have been shown to be correlated with prognosis in papillary carcinoma. Several studies have shown that in older patients papillary carcinoma behaves as a more aggressive tumour than in younger patients, and in the past it has been suggested that tumours arising before the age of 40 have a much better prognosis than tumours arising after the age of 40 (WOOLNER et al. 1961). The change in prognosis with age, however, appears to be continuous. Sex is also correlated with survival, males showing a slightly worse survival than females. It has also been shown that small primary tumours are associated with a better prognosis than large primary tumours, particularly those where the capsule of the gland is penetrated. The prognosis of a patient in whom all these factors are favourable is extremely good: a female patient with a small (less than 1.5 cm diameter) primary that has not involved the surface of the gland has a prognosis that is indistinguishable from normal. At the other extreme, an elderly male patient with a large primary papillary carcinoma spreading through the capsule of the thyroid has a relatively poor prognosis. Cervical lymph node involvement is common in patients with papillary carcinoma of the thyroid, and in the past it has been claimed that this is not correlated with any deterioration in prognosis; however, some doubt has been thrown on this recently (HARWOOD et al. 1978).

A number of enviromental factors have been known to influence the incidence of papillary carcinoma of the thyroid. There is little evidence that it is more common in goitrous areas; the reverse may well be true. In a selected series of papers showing the percentage distribution of thyroid carcinomas (BEAUGIE et al. 1976), the lowest percentage of papillary carcinoma was derived from a goitrois area. Papillary carcinoma has been shown to be unusually common in an iodide-rich area (WILLIAMS et al. 1977), and three separate studies from Switzerland have shown that papillary carcinoma has increased in frequency since the iodination of salt in that country (THALMANN 1954; HEITZ et al. 1976; BUBENDORFER and HEDINGER 1977). This evidence therefore suggests that papillary carcinoma may be more common in areas with high dietary iodide.

Microscopic papillary carcinomas are not uncommonly found at autopsy, their frequency depending in part upon the techniques used to study the thyroid. In one study, in which identical pathological techniques and diagnostic criteria were used, the prevalence of occult papillary carcinomas varied from 5.6% in Colombia to 28.4% in Japan. This variation may be related partly to the variation in dietary iodide intake, although the study did not show a correlation between gland size and tumour frequency (FUKUNAGA and YATANI 1975).

Radiation is clearly of considerable importance in the causation of thyroid carcinoma, and most radiation-induced tumours have been found to be papillary in type. It is nearly 30 years since the association of radiation of the neck in infancy with the development of thyroid tumours in later life was demonstrated (DUFFY and FITZGERALD 1950). The original observation has now been confirmed many times over, and studies on several thousand children irradiated for so-called thymic enlargement have shown a considerably higher incidence of thyroid carcinoma among them than among their nonirradiated siblings (HEMPELMANN 1969). External radiation given for a wide variety of reasons and over a wide dose range has been implicated in the genesis of papillary carcinoma of the thyroid. As well as "enlarged thymus", enlarged tonsils and adenoids, cervical lymphadenopathy due to tuberculosis or Hodgkin's disease, whooping cough, cerebral tumours, and a variety of skin conditions including angioma, keloid, acne vulgaris, and tinea capitis, have all been irradiated with subsequent development of thyroid tumours in some instances. Doses as low as 6.5 rads have been shown to increase the incidence of thyroid tumours in later life (MODAN et al. 1974). There is evidence that the incidence of thyroid carcinoma declines with doses above 2000 rads (HANFORD et al. 1962) and increases with doses between 100 and 600 rads (HEMPELMANN 1969). Radiation must therefore be accepted as an important aetiological factor in the genesis of papillary carcinoma of the thyroid, particularly in young people. A recent survey of over 2500 individuals who had had head and neck radiation for benign conditions showed that the probability of finding thyroid cancer in a nodular gland was increased in irradiated patients (SCHNEIDER et al. 1978). To maintain a perspective in this matter, however, it should be pointed out that the same survey found only one subject who was known to have died from thyroid carcinoma.

Thyroiditis has been implicated as a possible aetiological factor for papillary carcinoma in the past (HIRABAYASHI and LINDSAY 1965). It now seems more likely that in some instances the presence of the tumour stimulates an immune response, possibly through follicular disruption. In a comparative study of two areas with widely differing incidences of thyroiditis no correlation was found between papillary carcinoma and the presence of absence of thyroiditis (WILLIAMS et al. 1977). It seems unlikely that thyroiditis is an important aetiological factor for papillary carcinoma.

The role of racial and genetic factors in the genesis of papillary carcinoma is ill-defined. Papillary carcinoma has been described in patients with Gardner's syndrome (CAMIEL et al. 1968; SMITH and KERN 1973), and this link with multiple polyposis of the colon is perhaps not surprising in a gut-derived organ. It is not possible to disentangle environmental from racial and genetic influences in studies on the incidence of papillary carcinoma in different countries, quite apart from the problems that may result from the use of different techniques and diagnostic criteria in the study of these tumours.

Follicular Carcinoma

Follicular carcinoma is less common than papillary carcinoma in the great majority of published series. The range of percentage distribution of follicular carcinoma lies between about 10% and 40%. In the Mayo Clinic series (WOOLNER et al. 1961) it was found in a broad-age range, with a mean age at presentation of 50 – slightly higher than for papillary carcinoma. It can be subdivided into will-differentiated and moderately differentiated subgroups (HEDINGER and SOBIN 1974), the moderately differentiated group showing a poorer prognosis. As with papillary carcinoma, the prognosis worsens with increasing age at presentation and is slightly poorer for males than for females. These observations are true when the subgroups are examined separately (BYAR et al. [to be published]; WILLIAMS et al. [to be published]).

The relationship of follicular carcinoma to dietary iodide appears to be the obverse of that discussed for papillary carcinoma. The highest incidence of follicular carcinoma has been reported from goitrous areas (WAHNER et al. 1966; PERINETTI et al. 1974); the relative incidence of follicular carcinomas was extremely low in an iodide-rich area (WILLIAMS et al. 1977) and the incidence of follicular carcinoma has declined since the addition of iodide to the diet in Switzerland (THALMANN 1954; HEITZ et al. 1976; BUBENDORFER and HEDINGER 1977). The high incidence in goitrous areas and its reduction after iodination of the diet may well be related to the level of TSH. In dyshormonogenesis the prolonged high TSH that is a sequel to the biochemical defect impairing the efficiency of thyroid hormone production regularly leads to the production of multiple benign follicular tumours. The development of carcinoma is rare, but in most reported cases it seems to be follicular in type (MEDEIROS-NETO and OLIVIERA 1970; STANBURY 1969).

Radiation is also carcinogenic for follicular carcinoma, although as remarked above, the great bulk of radiation-induced tumours are papillary in type. Genetic factors are very rarely involved in the aetiology of follicular tumours, although follicular adenoma has been described in association with ovarian arrhenoblastoma and follicular tumours in the ill-defined entity of Cowden's syndrome (LLOYD and DENNIS 1963; WEARY et al. 1972).

Anaplastic Carcinoma

In most series anaplastic carcinoma makes up 5%–30% of thyroid carcinomas. Figures for its existence must be regarded with caution, however, not only because relative incidence figures may largely reflect the proportion of elderly people in the population, but also because in the past many malignant lymphomas have been included under this heading. In the Mayo Clinic series (WOOLNER et al. 1961) anaplastic carcinoma was not found in children; the mean age at presentation was 57 years, and the sex ratio (female : male) was 1.3 : 1. It is an extremely uncommon tumour below the age of 40, and is associated with an exceptionally poor prognosis, 60% of patients being dead within 6 months of the diagnosis. The evidence already quoted for the development of anaplastic carcinoma from pre-existing differentiated carcinoma suggests that in considering its aetiology one should consider the factors that are likely to transform a slowly into a rapidly growing tumour. Age must obviously be taken into account, although it is perhaps likely simply that longer life of a papillary of follicular carcinoma involves a greater likelihood of exposure to the "transforming agent". The high incidence of anaplastic carcinoma in Switzerland, compared with the United States of America (HEITZ et al. 1976), could be related to TSH stimulation, either through the increase in follicular carcinoma in the past, or through the effect of TSH on existing differentiated tumours. The very frequent diagnosis, in Switzerland, of malignant haemangio-endothelioma of the thyroid, originally considered a separate entity but now thought to be a variant of undifferentiated carcinoma (HEDINGER and SOBIN 1974), could also be due to the effect of raised TSH in an iodide-deficient area. It will be interesting to follow the incidence of both anaplastic carcinoma and malignant haemangio-endothelioma in Switzerland with increasing time after iodination.

Radiation must be considered of potential importance in the genesis of anaplastic carcinoma. There have been a number of individual case reports of this sequence. However, the very large cooperative study that compared the existence of thyroid cancer in patients treated for thyrotoxicosis by surgery, antithyroid drugs, or radioactive iodine failed to reach a definite conclusion (DOBYNS et al. 1974). In this study the glands removed by surgery revealed a number of unsuspected small cancers. It could therefore be argued that more tumours could be expected after radiation than after surgery, simply because they had not been removed by treatment. However, all five patients who died from anaplastic thyroid malignancy had received ^{131}I therapy, and no anaplastic carcinomas developed in patients treated by surgery or antithyroid drugs without radioiodine in this study. When the individual case reports of patients who have developed anaplastic carcinoma following radiation are examined, it can be seen that the age at which the tumour develops is much lower than that for most cases of anaplastic carcinoma. It seems reasonable to conclude that radiation is a rare cause of the development of anaplastic carcinoma of the thyroid in man.

A second possible factor to be considered is a virus-induced transformation. There is at present no direct evidence for this, and the suggestion could be regarded as personal speculation. However, the mechanisms that exist in normal cells for preventing virus-induced transformation may well be impaired in the cells of differentiated carcinoma.

While it seems likely that all anaplastic thyroid carcinomas arise from pre-existing differentiated thyroid carcinomas, it must be remembered that only a very small proportion of differentiated carcinomas will progress to anaplastic carcinomas. The proportion is so small that the possibility of anaplastic transformation is only of minor significance in determining the plan of treatment of differentiated thyroid carcinoma.

Medullary Carcinoma (MCT)

Medullary carcinoma accounts for 3%–10% of all thyroid carcinomas in most series (WILLIAMS 1975). It may present at almost any age, with a mean age of 49 years. The sex ratio (female : male) is 1.3 : 1 (WILLIAMS et al. 1966). Its growth rate varies widely; some tumours progress very slowly and survivals of 20–30 years are not uncommon. In contrast to papillary carcinoma, however, a high proportion of patients with medullary carcinoma eventually die from their tumour. Also in contrast to other types of thyroid malignancy, inheritance plays a major role in the aetiology of medullary carcinoma. As many as 20% of cases may be genetically mediated (CHONG et al. 1975; DUNN et al. 1973; GORDON et al. 1973). The figure is so high that it may in part account for the variation in relative incidence of medullary carcinoma in different series.

The tumour can be inherited as part of three distinct genetic syndromes, by itself, together with phaeochromocytoma, or as part of a complex syndrome with multiple mucosal neuromas, phaeochromocytomas, and many other abnormalities (WILLIAMS 1979). In each of these syndromes it is inherited as an autosomal dominant of very high penetrance. It has been shown over the past few years that the MCT in inherited syndromes is preceded by C-cell hyperplasia, and also that the phaeochromocytomas are preceded by adrenal medullary hyperplasia (WOLFE et al. 1973; CARNEY et al. 1976; DELELLIS et al. 1976). The natural history of the development of MCT therefore seems to begin with an abnormal stimulus (or an abnormal response to a normal stimulus) leading to diffuse hyperplasia of the C-cells, which in turn leads to the development of carcinoma.

There is some evidence that the degree of malignancy in the different syndromes may vary: in patients with multiple mucosal neuromas MCT presents at an earlier age and shows a higher degree of malignancy than MCT in some families with inherited MCT and phaeochromocytoma. No other significant factors are known to influence the incidence of MCT in man, although there are wide variations in its relative incidence in different series. Radiation has been reported as preceding the development of MCT in man in one case (DUNN et al. 1973) and also in an animal model of medullary carcinoma (TRIGGS and WILLIAMS 1977). The possibility that changes in dietary vitamin D or calcium may be important in the genesis of MCT in man remains to be investigated.

Malignant Lymphoma

Malignant lymphoma of the thyroid accounts for up to 12% of all types of thyroid malignancy. However, as with anaplastic carcinoma, the figures from different series have to be regarded with caution, partly because it too is a tumour that is largely confined to the elderly. The mean age at presentation in a recent series was 65, and it was not below 40 in any of the patients (BURKE et al. 1977). The survival is better in patients in whom the lymphoma is confined to the thyroid. The sex ratio is predominantly female, the ratio being approximately 3 : 1.

One of the most important observations relating to the aetiology of malignant lymphomas is that the great majority of cases where material is available for study show evidence of severe thyroiditis, often of the Hashimoto type (WOOLNER et al. 1961; WILLIAMS et al. 1977; BURKE et al. 1977). A comparative study of the existence of various types of thyroid malignancy in Iceland and Northeast Scotland showed that malignant lymphoma was more frequent in the area that also showed the higher incidence of thyroiditis in the population (WILLIAMS et al. 1977). A separate study showed that the incidence of circulating thyroid antibodies correlated with the frequency of thyroiditis (HEDLEY et al. 1977). It therefore seems reasonable to conclude that the severe thyroiditis found in many patients with malignant lymphoma of the thyroid is not a response to the tumour, but that the lymphoma arises from a pre-existing thyroiditis. This observation parallels the occurrence of malignant lymphoma of the parotid in patients with Sjogren's syndrome, and suggests that there may be a more general association of organ-specific malignant lymphoma with organ-specific autoimmune disease. However, in parallel to the remarks on anaplastic carcinoma, while most cases with malignant lymphoma show evidence of pre-existing thyroiditis, only a minute proportion of patients with thyroiditis develop malignant lymphoma. This link is not an argument for more radical treatment of thyroiditis in general. In a patient with proven thyroiditis and a markedly irregular or rapidly enlarging gland this diagnosis should be considered.

Conclusion

The main theme of this Chapter has been the demonstration that the pathology and natural history of thyroid cancer are inextricably linked. It is essential for any study in thyroid cancer that an accurate, reproducible, and generally acceptable classification should be used; this is now available through the World Health Organization's tumour pathology programme (HEDINGER and SOBIN 1974). The great majority of examples of thyroid cancer fall into five types, each with its characteristic natural history. The major aetiological factors known to be involved in the genesis of thyroid carcinoma do not affect the different subtypes equally. It is of particular interest that while follicular carcinoma appears to be more common in areas of iodide deficiency, the same it not true of papillary carcinoma, which is more common in areas of iodine excess. Radiation is of particular importance in the aetiology of papillary carcinoma, but may also be relevant for some cases of anaplastic carcinoma. Genetic influences are of particular importance in relation to medullary carcinoma, and thyroiditis is a significant factor in the aetiology of malignant lymphoma of the thyroid. It is hoped that any future study on the epidemiology of cancer of the thyroid will be firmly based on pathology.

References

1 Beaugie JM, Brown CL, Doniach I, Richardson JE (1976) Primary malignant tumours of the thyroid, the relationship between histological classification and clinical behaviour. Br J Surg 63:173–181
2 Bubendorfer R, Hedinger C (1977) Schilddrüsenmalignome vor und nach Einführung der Jodsalzprophylaxe. Schweiz Med Wochenschr 107:733–741
3 Burke JS, Butler JJ, Fuller LM (1977) Malignant lymphomas of the thyroid. Cancer 39:1587–1602
4 Byar DP, Green SB, Dor P, Williams ED, Colon J, van Gilse HJ, Sylvester R (to be published) A prognostic index for thyroid carcinoma. Eur J Cancer
5 Camiel MR, Mule JE, Alexander LL, Benninghoff DL (1968) Association of thyroid carcinoma with Gardner's syndrome in siblings. N Engl J Med 259:1056–1058
6 Carney JA, Sizemore GW, Sheps SG (1976) Adrenal medullary disease in multiple endocrine neoplasia, type 2. Am J Clin Pathol 66:279–290
7 Chong GC, Beahrs OH, Sizemore GW, Woolner LH (1975) Medullary carcinoma of the thyroid gland. Cancer 35:695–704
8 DeLellis RA, Wolfe JH, Gagel RF, Feldman ZT, Miller HH, Gang DL, Reichlin S (1976) Adrenal medullary hyperplasia. Am J Pathol 83:177–190

9 Dobyns BM, Sheline GE, Workman JB, Tompkins EA, McConahey WM, Becker DV (1974) Malignant and benign neoplasms of the thyroid in patients treated for hyperthyroidism: A report of the co-operative thyrotoxicosis therapy follow-up study. J Clin Endocrinol Metab 38:976–998
10 Duffy BJ, Fitzgerald PJ (1950) Cancer of the thyroid in children, a report of 28 cases. J Clin Endocrinol Metab 10:1296–1308
11 Dunn EL, Nishiyama RH, Thompson NW (1973) Medullary carcinoma of the thyroid gland. Surgery 73:848–858
12 Fukunaga FH, Yatani R (1975) Geographic pathology of occult thyroid carcinomas. Cancer 36:1095–1099
13 Gordon PR, Huvos AG, Strong EW (1973) Medullary carcinoma of the thyroid gland – a clinicopathologic study of 40 cases. Cancer 31:915–924
14 Hanford JM, Quimby EH, Frantz VK (1962) Cancer arising many years after radiation therapy. JAMA 181:404–410
15 Harwood J, Clark OH, Dunphy JE (1978) Significance of lymph node metastasis in differentiated thyroid cancer. Am J Surg 136:107–112
16 Hedinger CE, Sobin LH (1974) Histological typing of thyroid tumours, vol 11. International histological classification of tumours. World Health Organization, Geneva
17 Hedley AJ, Thjodlieffson B, Donald D, Beck JS, Crook SJ, Chesters MI, Hall R (1977) Thyroid function in normal subjects in Iceland and Northeast Scotland. Clin Endocrinol (Oxf) 7:377–382
18 Heitz P, Moser H, Staub J-J (1976) A study of 573 thyroid tumours and 161 autopsy cases observed over a thirty year period. Cancer 37:2329–2337
19 Hempelmann LH (1969) Risk of thyroid neoplasms after irradiation in childhood. Science 160:159–163
20 Hirabayashi RN, Lindsay S (1965) The relationship of thyroid carcinoma and chronic thyroiditis. Surg Gynecol Obstet 121:243–252
21 Ibanez ML, Russell WO, Albores-Saavedra J, Lampertico P, White EC, Clark RL (1966) Thyroid carcinoma – biologic behaviour and mortality. Cancer 19:1039–1052
22 Lloyd KM, Dennis M (1963) Cowden's disease: A possible new symptom complex with multiple system involvement. Ann Intern Med 48:136–142
23 Medeiros-Neto GA, Oliviera NRC (1970) Follicular adenocarcinoma of thyroid associated with congenital hyperplastic goiter. Acta Endocrinol Panam 1:73–89
24 Modan B, Baidatz D, Mart H, Steinitz R, Levin SG (1974) Radiation induced head and neck tumours. Lancet 1:277–279
25 Perinetti H, Staneloni LN, Yaciofano CA, Nora JN, Giner M, Tejeda JS, Perinetti HA (1979) Cancer tiroideo en una region de bocio endemico. La Plata
26 Schneider AB, Favus MJ, Stachura ME, Arnold J, Arnold MJ, Frohman LA (1978) Incidence, prevalence and characteristics of radiation-induced thyroid tumours. Am J Med 64:243–252
27 Smith WG, Kern BB (1973) The nature of the mutation in familial polyposis. Dis Colon Rectum 16:264–271
28 Stanbury JB (1969) Thyroid-specific metabolic incompetence and tumour development. In: Hedinger CE (ed) Thyroid cancer, vol 12 UICC monograph series. Springer, Berlin Heidelberg New York (UICC monograph series, vol 12, Springer, pp 183–190)
29 Thalmann A (1954) Die Häufigkeit der Struma maligna am Berner Pathologischen Institut von 1910–1950 und ihre Beziehung zur Jodprophylaxe des endemischen Kropfes. Schweiz Med Wochenschr 84:473–478
30 Triggs SM, Williams ED (1977) Experimental carcinogenesis in the rat thyroid follicular and C cells. Acta Endocrinol (Kbh) 85:84–92
31 Wahner HW, Cuello C, Correa P, Uribe LF, Gaitan E (1966) Thyroid carcinoma in an endemic goiter area, Cali, Colombia. Am J Med 40:58–66

32 Weary PE, Gorlin RJ, Gentry WC Jr, Comer JE, Greer KE (1972) Multiple hamartoma syndrome (Cowden's disease). Arch Dermatol 106:682–690
33 Williams ED (1975) Medullary carcinoma of the thyroid. In: Harrison CV, Weinbren K (eds) Recent advances in pathology, 9th edn. Churchill Livingstone, Edinburgh, pp 156–182
34 Williams ED (1979) Medullary carcinoma of the thyroid. In: DeGroot LJ (ed) Endocrinology: Metabolic basis of clinical practice, vol 2. Grune & Stratton, New York, pp 777–792
35 Williams ED, Brown CL, Doniach I (1966) Pathological and clinical findings in a series of 67 cases of medullary carcinoma of the thyroid. J Clin Pathol 19:103–113
36 Williams ED, Doniach I, Bjarnason O, Michie W (1977) Thyroid cancer in an iodide rich area. Cancer 39:215–222
37 Wolfe HJ, Melvin KEW, Cervi-Skinner SJ, Al Saadi AA, Juliar JF, Jackson CE, Tashjian AH (1973) C cell hyperplasia preceding medullary thyroid carcinoma. N Engl J Med 289:437–441
38 Woolner LB, Beahrs OH, Black BM, McConahey WM, Keating FR Jr (1961) Classification and prognosis of thyroid carcinoma. Am J Surg 102:354–387

Immunological Aspects of Thyroid Cancer

R. Hall, M. Ross, C. S. Teng, and B. Rees Smith

Royal Victoria Infirmary, GB-Newcastle-upon-Tyne

Introduction

The role of immunological factors in the pathogenesis of thyroid cancer is complex and poorly understood. In this review the immunological associations of thyroid cancer will be considered in relation to three clinical entities, autoimmune thyroid disease, Graves' disease, and thyroid lymphoma.

Autoimmune Thyroid Disease and Thyroid Cancer

There have been a series of reports both in favour and against an association of thyroid cancer and focal and diffuse thyroiditis, and these are well reviewed by DONIACH (1970). The problem can be viewed from several aspects:

1) Frequency of thyroid cancer in patients with Hashimoto's thyroiditis,
2) frequency of thyroiditis in patients with different types of thyroid cancer,
3) frequency of thyroglobulin and microsomal antibodies in patients with different types of thyroid cancer.

Thyroid Cancer in Patients with Hashimoto's Thyroiditis

The frequency of thyroid cancer in patients with thyroiditis is unlikely to be greater than that expected by chance in the normal population (WOOLNER et al. 1959). The problem is that patients with Hashimoto's disease who have some clinical suggestion of malignancy, e.g., asymmetry of the gland or failure of response to thyroid hormone, are more likely to be operated on, and a spurious association of thyroiditis and cancer may thus be observed. In population studies papillary carcinoma has been shown to be common in Iceland, but thyroiditis is commoner in Scotland (WILLIAMS et al. 1977).

Thyroiditis in Patients with Thyroid Cancer

The frequency of focal thyroiditis is probably higher in patients with thyroid cancer than in the general population (GOUDIE 1966), but this may well be due to local tissue damage produced by the tumour. The improved prognosis in papillary carcinomas accompanied by thyroiditis may be the result of reduced growth and metastases due to immunological factors.

Thyroglobulin and Microsomal Antibodies in Patients with Thyroid Cancer

There is controversy as to the frequency of thyroglobulin and microsomal antibodies in thyroid cancer. We have observed no increased prevalence of thyroglobulin and microsomal antibodies in 79 patients previously treated for thyroid cancer, whereas DeGroot et al. (1977), from the United States, reported an increase in both antibodies. The nature of the control population is obviously of great importance, and our comparison is based on a large age- and sex-matched normal population from the same area as the cancer patients (Tunbridge et al. 1977), whereas the source of the controls in DeGroot's series is not reported.

Graves' Disease and Thyroid Cancer

In animals, endogenous stimulation of the thyroid by thyroid-stimulating hormone (TSH) is associated with a clear increase in the incidence of thyroid cancer. In man, however, the situation is much less clear cut. The problem can be viewed from several aspects:

1) Frequency of thyroid cancer in patients with hyperthyroidism,
2) frequency of hyperthyroidism in patients with thyroid cancer,
3) frequency of thyroid-stimulating antibodies in patients with thyroid cancer,
4) frequency of Graves' ophthalmopathy in thyroid cancer.

Thyroid Cancer in Patients with Hyperthyroidism

Histological sections of 2114 thyroid glands from patients who had undergone partial thyroidectomy for hyperthyroidism were examined for evidence of thyroid cancer by Olen and Klinck (1966). In 53 instances a thyroid cancer was found, an incidence of 2.5%. Most of the cancers were small and more than half were of the occult sclerosing type of papillary carcinoma; 18 were papillary, five were follicular, and three were poorly differentiated. In only four patients had the carcinoma spread to regional lymph nodes. These findings can be compared with a frequency of 2.8% found by Mortensen et al. (1955) in 1000 consecutive routine autopsies, suggesting that there is no elevated frequency of carcinoma in glands removed for hyperthyroidism. However, the subjects in Mortensen's series were older, with fewer female patients, and the histological examination was more rigorous than in the series of Olen and Klinck (1966), which raises some doubt about a negative conclusion.

Hyperthyroidism in Patients with Thyroid Cancer

Hyperthyroidism is rare in patients with thyroid cancer. Valenta et al. (1969) found three definite cases of hyperthyroidism in a series of about 300 patients treated for thyroid cancer in Prague. However, it seems unlikely that all the cancer patients were actually reviewed for evidence of thyroid overactivity. This contrasts with incidences of 8.3% for hyperthyroidism in 120 cases of thyroid cancer reported from Sheffield (Hancock et al. 1977) and 3.8% in our own series of 79 patients. Obviously selection of patients as well as geographical factors must influence this discrepancy. The frequency of hyperthyroidism in the northeast of England is 2.7% in females, a value not significantly different from the 3.8% incidence of hyperthyroidism observed in our cancer series.

Thyroid-stimulating Antibodies in Patients with Thyroid Cancer

It is now accepted that thyroid-stimulating antibodies (TSAb) are the cause of the hyperthyroidism and goitre in Graves' disease (REES SMITH and HALL 1974; BROWN et al. 1978). They appear to be antibodies to the TSH receptor, which bind to the receptor and cause the activation of adenyl cyclase, though some antibodies bind without causing thyroid stimulation. TSAb can be detected by the McKenzie mouse bioassay, the activity in this system being referred to as long-acting thyroid stimulator (LATS), (CLAGUE et al. 1976) by a receptor assay (REES SMITH and HALL 1974) and by the LATS-protector (LATS-P) assay. VALENTA et al. (1969) detected LATS in three of their patients with hyperthyroidism and thyroid cancer, though HANCOCK et al. (1977) found LATS-P in only one in eight of their patients. FENZI et al. (1978) were unable to detect TSAb by receptor assay in 12 patients with thyroid cancer, whereas we have observed TSAb in 20% of 79 patients with a variety of types of thyroid cancer (ROSS et al. [to be published]). Reasons for these discrepancies could include differences in patient selection, assay procedures, geographical factors, and the effects of therapy. There is evidence that thyroid damage caused by viruses, as in subacute thyroiditis (STRAKOSCH et al. 1978), or by radioiodine (KRISS et al. 1966) can lead to TSAb production, and it remains possible that the TSAb we have detected could have resulted from thyroid damage induced by the tumour or by thyroidectomy, or from radiation. The biological activity of the TSAb measured by the receptor and LATS-P assays required confirmation. In our patient reported by SNOW et al. [to be published] the appearance of metastases from a follicular carcinoma of the thyroid appeared to coincide with the development of Graves' disease and TSAb.

Graves' Ophthalmopathy in Patients with Thyroid Cancer

Graves' ophthalmopathy has been reported to follow radiation to the neck for nonthyroidal neoplastic disease. In our series of 79 patients with thyroid cancer, six had ocular signs of Graves' disease, a frequency higher than would have been expected by chance (ROSS et al. [to be published]). It is possible that thyroid damage (see previous Section) could have contributed to the development of the ophthalmopathy, possibly as the result of release of antigens common to the thyroid and orbital tissue.

It seems unlikely, therefore, that there is any striking association between hyperthyroidism and thyoid cancer, but there is preliminary evidence for some association of TSAb and Graves' ophthalmopathy with thyroid cancer.

Lymphoma of the Thyroid and Thyroiditis

There is now good evidence for an increased frequency of thyroiditis and microsomal and thyroglobulin antibodies in patients with lymphoma of the thyroid. It therefore seems likely that thyroiditis is a predisposing factor to the malignancy, just as the immunological reactions in the parotid gland and thymus are associated with the lymphomas of Sjogren's syndrome and the thymomas of myasthenia gravis, respectively. Thyroid lymphomas have long been known to be associated with lymphomas of the gastrointestinal tract (BREWER and ORR 1953), but it is now realized that thyroid lymphoma may merely be a local manifestation of a more general lymphomatous process.

References

1. Brewer DB, Orr JW (1953) Struma reticulosa: A reconsideration of the undifferentiated tumours of the thyroid. J Pathol Bact 65:193–208
2. Brown RS, Jackson IMD, Pohl SL, Reichlin S (1978) Do thyroid-stimulating immunoglobulins cause non-toxic and toxic multinodular goitre? Lancet 1:904–906
3. Clague R, Mukhtar ED, Pyle GA, Nutt J, Clark F, Scott M, Evered D, Rees Smith B, Hall R (1976) Thyroid-stimulating immunoglobulins and control of thyroid function. J Clin Endocrinol Metab 43:550–555
4. DeGroot LJ, Haye K, Refetoff S, Van Herle AJ, Asteris GT, Rochman H (1977) Serum antigens and antibodies in the diagnosis of thyroid cancer. J Clin Endocrinol. Metab 45:1220–1223
5. Doniach I (1970) Aetiological consideration of thyroid carcinoma. In: Smithers D (ed) Tumours of the thyroid gland. Livingstone, Edinburgh London, pp 55–72
6. Fenzi G, Macchia E, Bartalena L, Mazzanti F, Baschieri L, DeGroot LJ (1978) Radio-receptor assay of TSH: its use to detect thyroid-stimulating immunoglobulins. J Endocrinol Invest 1:17124
7. Goudie RB (1966) Thyroiditis and thyroid carcinoma, In: Appaix A (ed) Tumours of the thyroid gland. Karger, Basel New York, p 292
8. Hancock BW, Bing RF, Dirmikis SM, Munro DS, Neal FE (1971) Thyroid carcinoma and concurrent hyperthyroidism. A study of ten patients. Cancer 39:298–302
9. Kriss JP, Pleshakov V, Chien JR (1964) Isolation and identification of the long-acting thyroid stimulator and its relation to hyperthyroidism and circumscribed pretibial myxoedema. J Clin Endocrinol Metab 24:1005–1028
10. Mortensen JD, Bennett WA, Woolner LB (1955) Incidence of carcinoma in thyroid glands removed at 1000 consecutive routine necropsies. Sing Forum 5:659–663
11. Olen E, Klinck GH (1966) Hyperthyroidism and thyroid cancer. Arch Pathol 81:531–535
12. Rees Smith B, Hall R (1974) Thyroid-stimulating immunoglobulins in Graves' disease. Lancet 2:427–431
13. Ross WM, Teng CS, Davies TF, Scanlon MF, Evered DC, Rees Smith B, Hall R (to be published) Thyroid-stimulating antibodies, Graves' disease and thyroid cancer. J Clin Endocrinol Metab
14. Snow MF, Davies T, Rees Smith B, Ross WM, Evans RGB, Teng CS, Hall R (to be published) Thyroid-stimulating antibodies and metastic thyroid carcinoma. J Clin Endocrinol Metab
15. Strakosch CR, Joyner D, Wall JR (1978) Thyroid-stimulating antibodies in patients with subacute thyroiditis. J Clin Endocrinol Metab 46:345–348
16. Tunbridge WMG, Evered DC, Hall R, Appleton D, Brewis M, Clark F, Grimley Evans J, Young E, Bird T, Smith PA (1977) The spectrum of thyroid disease in a community: the Whickham Survey. J Clin Endocrinol Metab 7:481–493
17. Valenta L, Lemarchand-Berand T, Nemec J, Griessen M, Bednar J (1969) Metastic thyroid carcinoma provoking hyperthyroidism, with elevated circulating thyrostimulators. Am J Med 48:72–76
18. Williams ED, Doniach I, Bjarnason O, Michie W (1977) Thyroid cancer in an iodide rich area Cancer 39:215–222
19. Woolner LB, McConahey WM, Beahrs OH (1959) Struma lymphomatosa (Hashimoto's thyroiditis) and related thyroidal disorders. J Clin Endocrinol Metab 19:53–57

Tumour Markers

J. C. Stevenson and C. J. Hillyard

Endocrine Unit, Royal Postgraduate Medical School, Ducane Road, GB-London W12 OHS

Introduction

The primary use of a tumour marker is to indicate the presence of a tumour. It can therefore be used to screen people who are known to be at high risk of developing the tumour. It can be used to demonstrate dissemination of a tumour, in which case it is an aid to the management of the patient. It can be used both to monitor treatment and to detect any recurrence of the disease at the earliest possible stage. The practical importance of such a marker depends on the frequency of its occurrence in patients with the tumour. There should be a good correlation between the peripherally measured level of the marker and the actual mass of tumour cells. Furthermore, effective treatment for the tumour must be available.

In patients with medullary carcinoma of the thyroid, the hormone calcitonin fulfils these criteria and is thus an ideal tumour marker for this condition.

Historical Background

Medullary thyroid carcinoma (MCT) was recognised as a distinct clinical entity in 1959 (HAZARD et al. 1959), but its histological origin was not recognised until 1966, when WILLIAMS suggested that it was a tumour of the thyroid parafollicular cells (WILLIAMS 1966). These cells, now known as C cells (PEARSE 1966), are derived from the neural crest and secrete a peptide hormone called calcitonin.

This hormone was discovered by virtue of its calcium-lowering property (COPP et al. 1962) and was shown to originate from the thyroid gland by MACINTYRE and his colleagues (FOSTER et al. 1964). Circulating levels of this hormone can be measured by radioimmunoassay (CLARK et al. 1969), and in normal man they are extremely low.

The occurrence of MCT may be sporadic or familial. In both situations, measurement of plasma calcitonin is essential to diagnosis and management.

Sporadic MCT

This tumour is always associated with raised calcitonin levels (CUNLIFFE et al. 1968; TASHJIAN and MELVIN 1968; HILLYARD et al. 1975). These levels may be extremely high, reaching over 1 mg/litre in some cases. With extreme elevation of circulating calcitonin levels, the diagnosis of medullary thyroid carcinoma can usually be made with confidence, but a variety of nonthyroid tumours may be associated with elevated levels of plasma calcitonin,

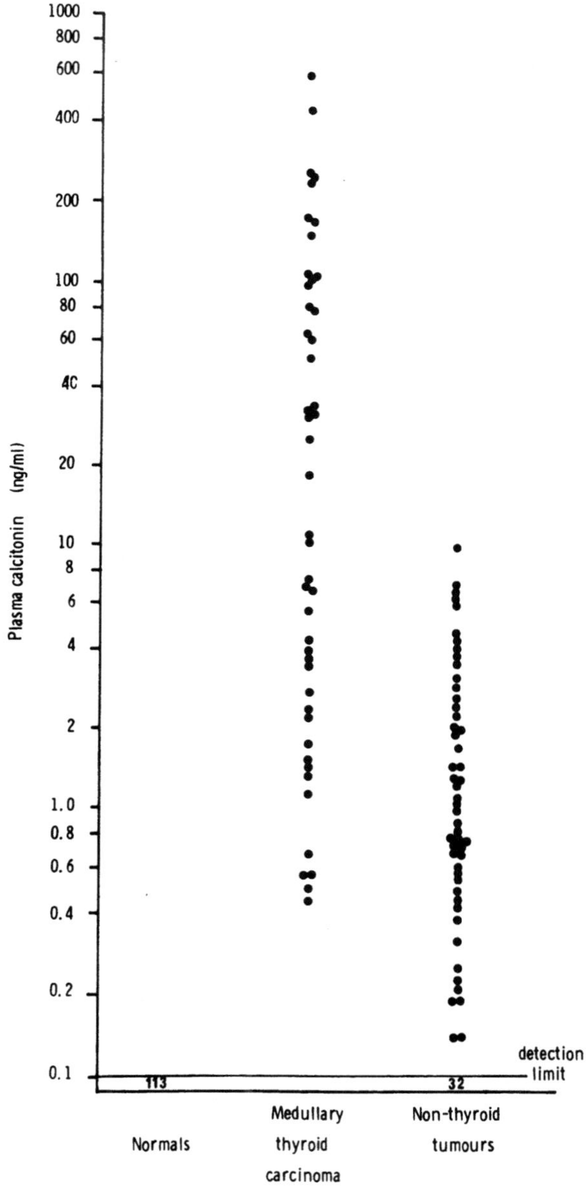

Fig. 1. Comparison of plasma calcitonin levels in normal subjects, patients with MCT, and patients with nonthyroid tumours

usually in the lower range of levels found with sporadic medullary carcinomas (COOMBES et al. 1974), as shown in Fig. 1.

The raised levels of plasma calcitonin found in some patients with nonthyroid neoplasms may be due either to ectopic secretion of the hormone by the tumour or to stimulation of the C cells by some unknown mechanism (SILVA et al. 1975). Mild elevation of plasma calcitonin may be found in patients with hypercalcaemia (CLARK et al. 1969). It has also been reported to occur in patients with primary hyperparathyroidism and in patients with hyperparathyroidism secondary to renal failure (HEYNEN and FRANCHIMONT 1974).

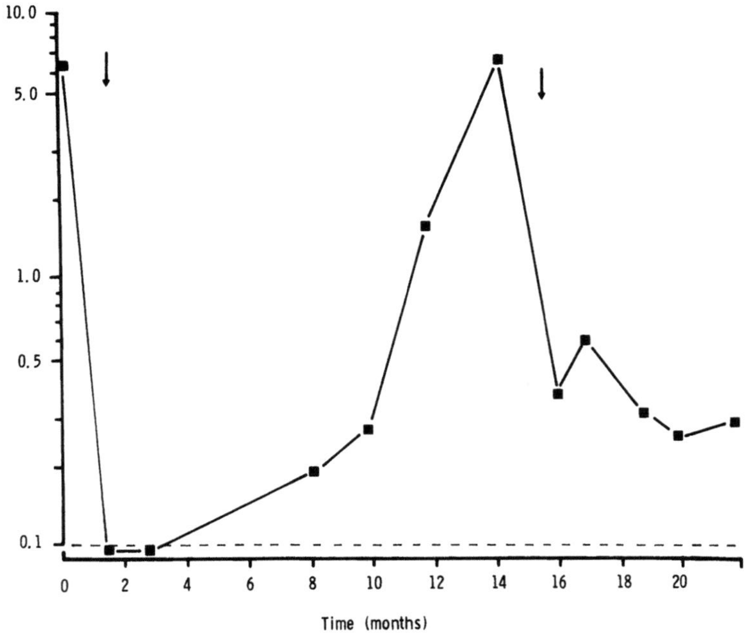

Fig. 2. Plasma calcitonin levels (ng/ml) measured during followup of a patient with sporadic MCT. *Broken horizontal line* indicates detection limit. *Arrows* indicate thyroidectomy (*left*) and removal of local metastasis (*right*)

Serial calcitonin measurements are used in postoperative follow-up of patients who have undergone thyroidectomy for medullary carcinoma (Fig. 2). A rise in circulating calcitonin levels will indicate recurrence of the disease and usually precedes the onset of clinical symptoms. In cases of recurrent disease or incomplete surgical treatment a neck localisation study may be performed. The neck veins are catheterised, venous samples are taken, and calcitonin levels are then estimated. An elevation of calcitonin in one particular vein may thus guide the surgeon to the site of recurrence (Fig. 3).

Familial MCT

The familial form of MCT is usually bilateral, and it has an autosomal dominant mode of inheritance (Schimke and Hartmann 1965). It may occur in association with other tumours as part of the multiple endocrine adenomatosis syndromes (Steiner et al. 1968; Block et al. 1975).

In this familial form calcitonin levels tend to be lower than in sporadic cases, and a small but significant number of patients have basal levels of the hormone that are within normal limits (Deftos 1974). In addition, calcitonin secretion by the tumour may be only intermittently abnormal, and thus circulating levels can fluctuate from day to day. Some of the cases with normal basal levels have only hyperplasia or early neoplasia of the C cells and provocative tests to stimulate calcitonin secretion are necessary for identification of these patients.

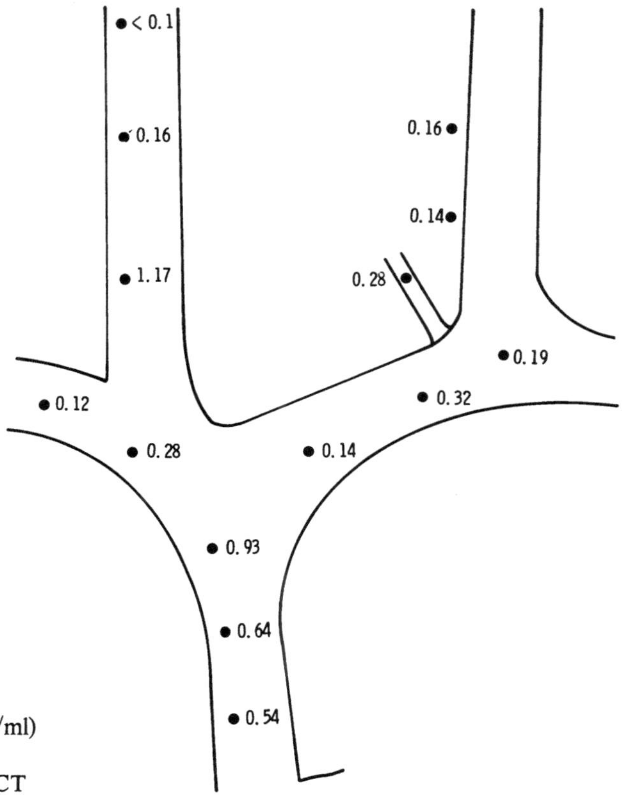

Fig. 3. Plasma calcitonin levels (ng/ml) found during selective venous catheterization of a patient with MCT

Provocative Tests

There are three agents in common use for provocative tests designed to identify patients with familial MCT accompanied by normal basal levels of calcitonin.

Calcium

It is well known that an IV calcium infusion can be used to stimulate calcitonin release in patients with MCT (CUNLIFFE et al. 1968; TASHJIAN et al. 1970). The standard infusion is over 4 h but it is associated with side effects such as hypertension and nausea. This test becomes impractical when large numbers of patients have to be screened.
Short infusions of calcium over 10 min (PARTHEMORE et al. 1974) or even 1 min (RUDE and SINGER 1977) have been found to be effective, but again side effects are frequent (WELLS et al. 1978).

Pentagastrin

Pentagastrin given as an IV bolus is another effective calcitonin secretagogue. There are conflicting reports of its efficacy compared with IV calcium (HENNESSEY et al. 1974; TELENIUS-BERG 1976; RUDE and SINGER 1977; WELLS et al. 1978). It usually produces a rapid and in-

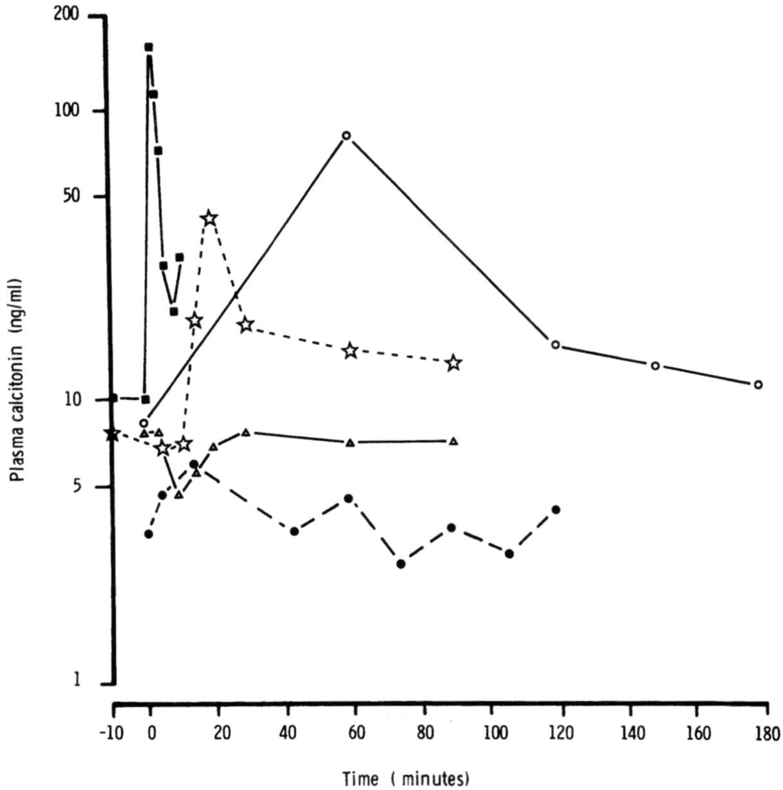

Fig. 4. Comparison of provocative tests in a woman patient with sporadic MCT. ■ – ■, 0.5 μg pentagastrin/kg body wt. IV; ○ – ○, 15 mg/Calcium/kg in isotonic saline IV over 3 h; ☆ – ☆ 50 ml oral whisky; △ – △, 50 ml oral water; ● – ●, 250 ml 15% ethanol IV over 1.50 h

tense rise in plasma calcitonin. However, the frequent side effects of retrosternal and abdominal pain and nausea have led us to limit the use of pentagastrin.

Alcohol

A major development in calcitonin stimulation occurred when a patient with MCT reported flushing and diarrhoea on drinking alcohol (Cohen et al. 1973). Oral alcohol was subsequently shown to be an effective calcitonin secretagogue (Dymling et al. 1976). It causes a fairly rapid rise in circulating calcitonin and is relatively free of unpleasant side effects compared with the other agents. In over 100 whisky tests analysed by our Unit there has always been a rise in plasma calcitonin in patients with initially elevated basal levels.

We use a standard oral dose of 50 ml 70° proof spirit (40% ethanol by volume) in adults and 30 ml in children. It should be drunk rapidly. Venous blood is collected into cooled, heparinised tubes basally, and at 3, 10, 15, and 30 min. The plasma must be separated immediately and stored at –20° C until assayed.

The mode of action of alcohol on calcitonin secretion remains unknown (Wells et al. 1975), but it may be mediated via adrenergic stimulation.

Other Agents

Cholecystokinin (TELENIUS-BERG 1976) and glucagon have been used as provocative agents. However, they have been found to be unsatisfactory because of variability in response or of side effects.
It has recently been suggested that a combination of IV calcium and pentagastrin is the most reliable stimulus for calcitonin secretion (WELLS et al. 1978). False-negative results have been reported with both calcium and pentagastrin (GAGEL et al. 1975), and much larger studies would be needed to support this conclusion, including comparison with oral alcohol. A comparison of all the major provocative agents is shown in Fig. 4. Oral alcohol compares favourably with other agents. Its relative lack of side effects and easy administration make it, in our experience, the provocative test of choice for screening for MCT. Obviously the timing and technique of collection of samples are important to prevent false-negative results.

Other Markers

Medullary thyroid carcinomas produce a variety of bioactive substances besides calcitonin. Two other possible markers have been studied in patients with these tumours.

Histaminase

Serum histaminase activity has been found to be increased in some patients with medullary thyroid carcinoma (BAYLIN et al. 1972). It is more usually raised in patients with metastatic disease and tends to be normal in patients with localised disease.

Carcinoembryonic Antigen (CEA)

Elevated peripheral levels of CEA have been reported in patients with both local and metastatic MCT (DELELLIS et al. 1978). In the same study, it was found that tumour cells generally contained immunoreactive CEA whereas normal and hyperplastic C cells did not.
Neither serum histaminase nor serum CEA has any advantage over calcitonin as a marker for medullary thyroid carcinoma; nor are they reliable for early detection of the disease.

Conclusions

Calcitonin is a most useful tumour marker in MCT. The measurement of circulating levels allows detection of the disease and, in familial cases, can distinguish family members who bear the gene. It can be used to monitor treatment of the disease and to detect recurrence at an early stage. In conjunction with neck localisation studies, it may help to indicate the site of recurrence of the disease if this occurs after thyroidectomy.

Provocative testing may be necessary to identify patients with early C-cell neoplasia or hyperplasia when basal calcitonin levels are normal. Alcohol is a simple, safe, and effective provocative agent that can be used for widespread screening for MCT.

Acknowledgements. This work was supported in part by the Arthritis and Rheumatism Council and the Cancer Research Campaign.

References

1 Baylin SB, Beaven MA, Keiser HR (1972) Serum histaminase and calcitonin levels in medullary carcinoma of the thyroid. Lancet 1:455–458

2 Block MB, Roberts JP, Kadair RF, Seyfer AE, Hull SF, Nofeldt FD (1975) Multiple endocrine adenomatosis type IIb. JAMA 234:710–714

3 Clark MB, Boyd GW, Byfield PGH, Foster GV (1969) A radioimmunoassay for human calcitonin M. Lancet 2:74–77

4 Cohen SL, MacIntyre I, Grahame-Smith D, Walker JG (1973) Alcohol-stimulated calcitonin release in medullary carcinoma of the thyroid. Lancet 2:1172–1174

5 Coombes RC, Hillyard C, Greenberg PB, MacIntyre I (1974) Plasma-immunoreactive-calcitonin in patients with non-thyroid tumours. Lancet 1:1080–1083

6 Copp DH, Cameron EC, Cheney BA, Davidson AGF, Henze KG (1962) Evidence for calcitonin – a new hormone from the parathyroid that lowers blood calcium. Endocrinology 70:638–649

7 Cunliffe WJ, Blade MM, Hall R, Johnstone IDA, Hodgson P, Shuster S, Gudmundsson TV, Joplin GF, Williams ED, Woodhouse NJY, Galante L, MacIntyre I (1968) A calcitonin-secreting thyroid tumour. Lancet 2:63–66

8 Deftos LJ (1974) Radioimmunoassay for calcitonin in medullary thyroid carcinoma. JAMA 227:403–406

9 DeLellis RA, Rule AH, Spiler I, Nathanson L, Tashjian AH, Wolfe HJ (1978) Calcitonin and carcinoembryonic antigen as tumor markers in medullary thyroid carcinoma. Am J Clin Pathol 70:587–594

10 Dymling JF, Ljungberg O, Hillyard CJ, Greenberg PB, Evans IMA, MacIntyre I (1976) Whisky: a new provocative test for calcitonin secretion. Acta Endocrinol (Kbh) 82:500–509

11 Foster GV, Baghdiantz A, Kumar MA, Slack E, Soliman HA, MacIntyre I (1964) Thyroid origin of calcitonin. Nature 202:1303–1305

12 Gagel RF, Melvin KEW, Tashjian AH, Miller HH, Feldman ZT, Wolfe HJ, DeLellis RA, Cerviskinner S, Reichlin S (1975) Natural history of the familial medullary thyroid carcinoma – pheochromocytoma syndrome and the identification of preneoplastic stages by screening studies: a five-year report. Trans Assoc Am Physicians 88:177–191

13 Hazard JB, Hawk WA, Crile G (1959) Medullary (solid) carcinoma of the thyroid – a clinicopathologic entity. J Clin Endocrinol Metab 19:152–161

14 Hennessey JF, Wells SA, Ontjes DA, Cooper CW (1974) A comparison of pentagastrin injection and calcium infusion as provocative agents for the detection of medullary carcinoma of the thyroid. J Clin Endocrinol Metab 39:487–495

15 Heynen G, Franchimont P (1974) Human calcitonin radioimmunoassay in normal and pathological conditions. Eur J Clin Invest 4:213–222

16 Hillyard CJ, Greenberg PB, Coombes RC, MacIntyre I, Ljungberg O, Dymling JF (1975) Applications of a radioimmunoassay for human calcitonin. In: Pasternak CA (ed) Radioimmunoassay in clinical biochemistry. Heyden, London, pp 245–252

17 Parthemore JG, Bronzert D, Roberts G, Deftos LJ (1974) A short calcium infusion in the diagnosis of medullary thyroid carcinoma. J Clin Endocrinol Metab 39:108–111

18 Pearse AGE (1966) The cytochemistry of the thyroid C cells and their relationship to calcitonin. Proc R Soc Lond [Biol] 164:478–487
19 Rude RK, Singer FR (1977) Comparison of serum calcitonin levels after a 1-minute calcium injection and after pentagastrin injection in the diagnosis of medullary thyroid carcinoma. J Clin Endocrinol Metab 44:980–983
20 Schimke RN, Hartmann WH (1965) Familial amyloid-producing medullary carcinoma and phaeochromocytoma. Ann Intern Med 63:1027–1039
21 Silva OL, Becker KL, Doppman JL, Snider RH, Moore CF (1975) Calcitonin levels in thyroid-vein blood of man. Am J Med Sci 269:37–41
22 Steiner AL, Goodman AD, Powers SR (1968) Study of a kindred with phaeochromocytoma, medullary thyroid carcinoma, hyperparathyroidism and Cushing's disease: multiple endocrine neoplasia type 2. Medicine (Baltimore) 47:371–409
23 Tashjian AH, Melvin KEW (1968) Medullary carcinoma of the thyroid gland. N Engl J Med 279:279–283
24 Tashjian AH, Howland BG, Melvin KEW, Hill CS (1970) Immunoassay of human calcitonin. N Engl J Med 283:890–895
25 Telenius-Berg M (1976) Diagnostic studies in medullary carcinoma of the thyroid. Acta Med Scand [Suppl] 596:1–59
26 Wells SA, Cooper CW, Ontjes DA (1975) Stimulation of thyrocalcitonin secretion by ethanol in patients with medullary thyroid carcinoma – an effect apparently not mediated by gastrin. Metabolism 24:1215–1219
27 Wells SA, Baylin SB, Linehan WM, Farrell RE, Cox EB, Cooper CW (1978) Provocative agents and the diagnosis of medullary carcinoma of the thyroid gland. Ann Surg 188:139–141
28 Williams ED (1966) Histogenesis of medullary carcinoma of the thyroid. J Clin Pathol 19:114–118

Nuclear Medicine in the Assessment of Thyroid Cancer

M. N. Maisey and S. Ng Tang Fui

Department of Nuclear Medicine, Guy's Hospital, GB-London, SE1 9RT

Introduction

Nuclear medicine is the application of radionuclides to the investigation and treatment of disease. In its widest form, the speciality of nuclear medicine is thus involved in the management and treatment of patients with thyroid cancer at all stages. For the purpose of this review, however, the discussion will be restricted to the investigation of thyroid cancer before and after treatment; the subject of radioiodine therapy will be dealt with elsewhere. There are two distinct applications, which will be dealt with separately: (1) Preoperative diagnosis, which is usually the investigation of the solitary thyroid nodule; (2) Postoperative assessment of residual functioning thyroid tissue and detection of residual or recurrent functioning tumour, including metastatic deposits.

Preoperative Diagnosis of Thyroid Cancer

We can consider five important clinical situations in which the possibility of thyroid malignancy may arise.

1) A solitary thyroid nodule found on palpation,
2) previous exposure of the head, neck, or upper thorax to ionizing radiation,
3) a multinodular goitre with clinical features that arouse suspicion,
4) rarely, local symptons such as hoarseness, dysphagia, or pain in the absence of an abnormal thyroid on palpation,
5) cervical lymphadenopathy or distant metastases when the primary source is unknown.

Solitary Thyroid Nodule

The prominent place assumed by the solitary thyroid nodule in any discussion on thyroid cancer is due to the fact that thyroid cancer most often presents as a solitary thyroid nodule, although the majority of solitary thyroid nodules are benign lesions such as colloid nodules, adenomas, or cysts. Owing to the frequency of solitary thyroid nodules as a clinical problem, it is not practical or necessary to remove every one that is encountered to exclude malignancy. Perlmutter and Slater (1956) found single thyroid nodules in 12% of routine autopsies (50% more than one nodule), about 20% of which were larger than 1 cm and might therefore be expected to be palpable or demonstrable on radionuclide scan if medical attention was

Table 1. Radionuclides used in thyroid scanning

	Energy (KeV)	β Particles	Half-life
^{131}I	364	Present	8 days
^{125}I	27	0	57 days
$^{99}Tc^{m}$	140	0	6 h
^{123}I	160	0	13 h

sought. Of course, many thyroid nodules are not diagnosed during life. The incidence of malignancy in this unselected series of solitary thyroid nodules was about 10%, but in clinical practice the observed incidence is modified by a number of factors, such as the frequency with which solitary thyroid nodules are diagnosed or the selection of patients for surgery. Thus, assuming the desirability of treating thyroid cancer (Beierwaltes 1978), a desirable aim is to detect as many cancers as possible. The function of investigations, of which the radionuclide thyroid scan is the most important, is therefore to allow one to be so nearly certain that a nodule is malignant that surgical treatment becomes essential, or to be so confident that cancer is not present that excision is considered unnecessary.

The Thyroid Scan

The choice of radionuclides used in thyroid imaging has been reviewed elsewhere (Goolden et al. 1968). The radionuclides and their principle characteristics are shown in Table 1. Technitium^{99m} pertechnetate ($^{99}Tc^{m}$) is the radionuclide currently most widely used for routine thyroid imaging, although many centres still use ^{131}I. However, ^{123}I with its ideal physical characteristics (Wellmann and Anger 1971) and its properties as a physiological tracer, is now being used more widely, the current limiting factors being availability and expense. The optimal method for thyroid scanning at present is as follows (Hurley et al. 1971; Ng Tang Fui and Maisey [to be published]):

$^{99}Tc^{m}$ Pertechnetate 2–5 mCi is injected IV. Pertechnetate secreted in the saliva is washed down with a drink of water immediately before imaging is commenced 20–30 min after the injection. A gamma camera fitted with a pinhole collimator is used; this has been shown to be superior to the rectilinear scanner (Hurley et al. 1971; Ryo et al. 1976).

The patient lies supine with the neck partially extended and the collimator positioned at a distance to provide maximum magnification: 100000 counts are collected and the image is recorded on to X-ray film. With a dedicated minicomputer interfaced to the gamma camera the $^{99}Tc^{m}$ pertechnetate uptake can be computed reliably and rapidly (Fig. 1).

It may be necessary to evaluate suspicious areas by further oblique views (Karelitz and Richards 1975) and by marking palpable nodules for full evaluation. With this technique thyroid nodules down to 0.8 cm can usually be identified (Maisey et al. 1973).

Use in the Diagnosis of Thyroid Cancer. There are four important results a thyroid scan may show when a clinically solitary thyroid nodule is investigated.

1) A solitary nonfunctioning or hypofunctioning nodule (i.e., "cold" nodule),
2) a functioning nodule (i.e., "hot" nodule),

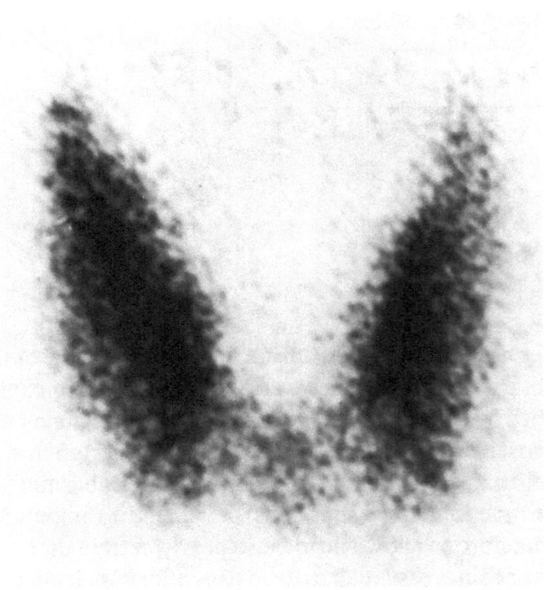

Fig. 1. Normal thyroid scan

3) a multinodular goitre,
4) a normal variant, or a normal thyroid with no evidence of an intrathyroidal nodule.

Solitary Cold Nodule. The probability of thyroid cancer is increased if a solitary cold nodule is found on the scan, but decreased considerably if any of the alternatives is observed. The incidence of thyroid cancer in solitary cold nodules has recently been reviewed by COWAN (1976) in 1252 patients from 13 reported series, and varies from 7% to 43% with an average of 19%, which is almost twice the average incidence of malignancy in unselected clinically solitary nodules, previously reported by PERLMUTTER and SLATER (1956). The probability of cancer in a solitary cold nodule is further increased if ultrasound examination is carried out and a solid lesion is demonstrated (Fig. 2), while if a cyst is found, as occurs with 20% of solitary cold nodules (MISKIN et al. 1973), the risk of malignancy if considerably reduced. About 1%–3% of cystic nodules are malignant (MA and ONG 1975), and this refers almost entirely to lesions that do not disappear completely after aspiration or that recur.

Hot Nodule. The finding of a functioning nodule in a euthyroid patient (Fig. 3), accounts for about 10% of all cases of solitary nodules (ALDERSON et al. 1976), makes the probability of carcinomas extremely low (PSARRAS et al. 1972) However, occasional cases have been reported in which the nodules are functioning on the pertechnetate scan but nonfunctioning on the iodine scan (MASSIN et al. 1977); this probably reflects the ability of the nodule to trap but not organify. Therefore, we routinely do a TRH test on any patient with a nodule that concentrates pertechnetate, as an absent TSH response to TRH confirms the nodule to be truly functioning and autonomous (Fig. 3). We only proceed to a radioiodine scan if the TRH test is normal, to eliminate the rare possibility of a disparity between pertechnetate and iodine. Naturally the more widespread use of ^{123}I will make this sequence unnecessary. There have also been a few case reports of thyroid cancer associated with hot nodules, but most, if not all

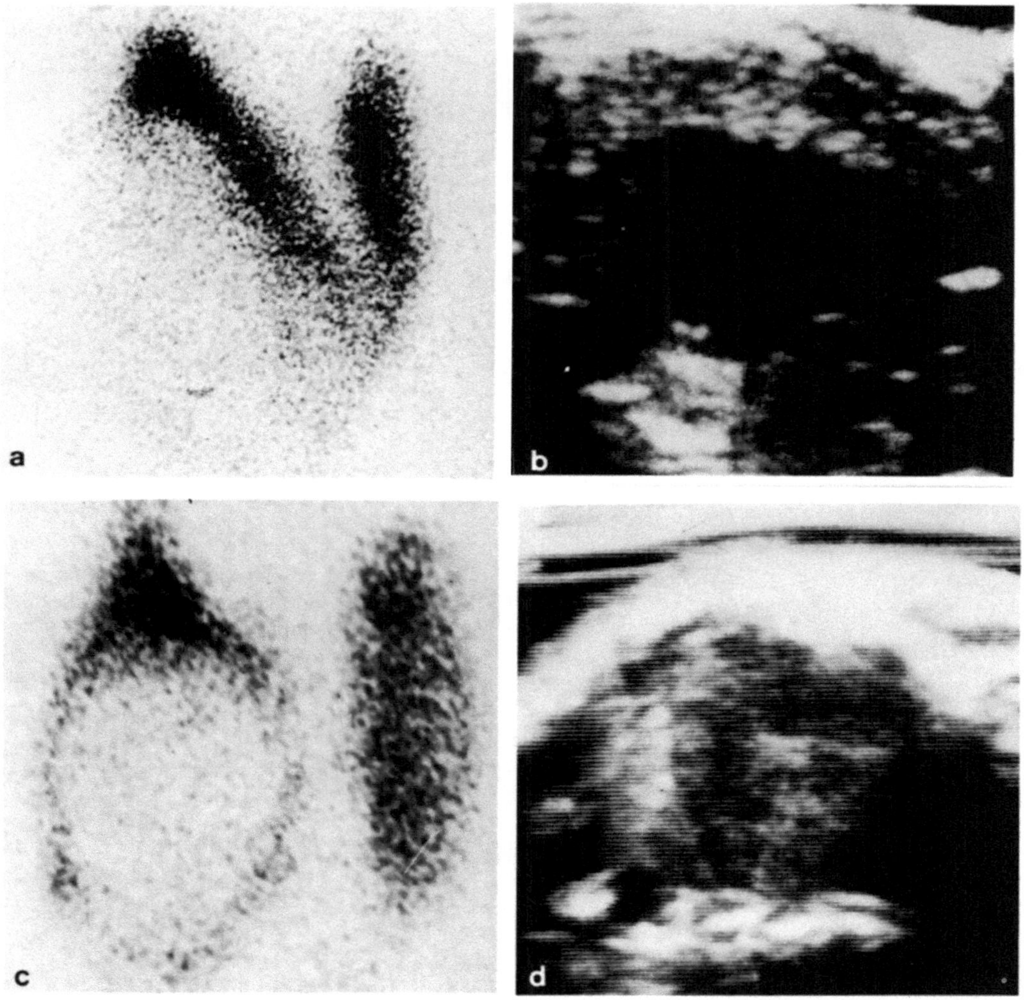

Fig. 2a–d. Ultrasound scan of solitary cold nodule. **a** $^{99}Tc^{m}$ scan; **b** ultrasound scan showing cyst; **c** $^{99}Tc^{m}$ scan; **d** ultrasound scan showing solid tumour

of the so-called malignant hot nodules were in fact cold malignant nodules adjacent to functioning nodules (WOLFSTEIN 1978).

Multinodular Goitre. The finding of a multinodular goitre when a solitary nodule has been suspected clinically also decreases the probability of thyroid cancer in the absence of other clinical evidence for malignancy. Approximately 36% of clinically diagnosed solitary thyroid nodules are shown to be multiple on scan (ALDERSON et al. 1976), and an even higher percentage at operation or autopsy (PERLMUTTER and SLATER 1956; MAISEY et al. 1973). Probably < 1% of multinodular goitres are malignant (LAHEY 1953), although in surgical series the incidence is about 3%–10% (PERLMUTTER and SLATER 1956; ANDERSON et al. 1976). This is because of the highly selective nature of surgical series. The presence of a dominant cold nodule in a gland with generally irregular uptake on the scan may increase the probability of malignancy (ALDERSON et al. 1976).

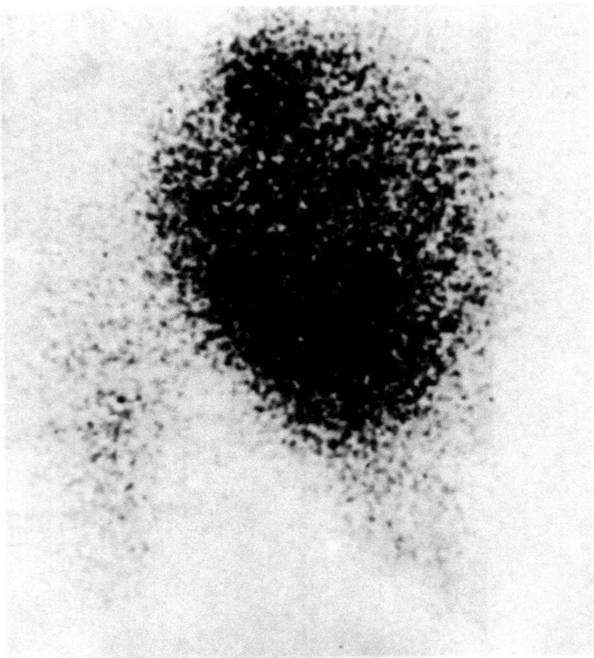

Fig. 3. Thyroid scan showing an autonomous hot nodule in the right lobe, with suppression of the rest of the gland

Table 2. Investigation of solitary thyroid nodule

Clinically solitary nodule —Thyroid scan→
- Hot nodule 10% —TRH test→
  - Normal →Radioiodine scan
  - Flat →Treat as hot nodule
- Multinodular 36%
  - Hot nodules
  - Simple multinodular
  - Dominant cold nodule
- Cold nodule 54% — Ultrasound
  - Cystic (20%)
  - Solid (80%)

The Normal Variant. Occasionally patients who are thought on clinical examination to have a thyroid nodule are shown by a scintigram to have a prominent, otherwise normal, lobe on the same side or the scan indicates that the palpable nodule is extrathyroidal.

As a result of these findings, we recommend the scheme shown in Table 2 for the investigation of the solitary thyroid nodule. The result of the scan should not be allowed to override clinical

Table 3. Other methods of investigating solitary thyroid nodules

1.	^{75}Selenomethionine scan (WEINSTEIN et al. 1971)
2.	^{67}Gallium citrate scan (KAPLAN et al. 1974; KOUTRAS et al. 1976)
3.	^{131}Caesium scan (KOUTRAS et al. 1976)
4.	^{201}Thallium scan (FUKUCHI et al. 1978)
5.	Needle biopsy: Core biopsy or aspiration cytology (WANG et al. 1976; GALVAN 1977)
6.	Fluorescent excitation analysis (PATTON et al. 1976)
7.	Computerised tomography (MEYBIER et al. 1978)
8.	Serum thyroglobulin (VAN HERLE et al. 1975)

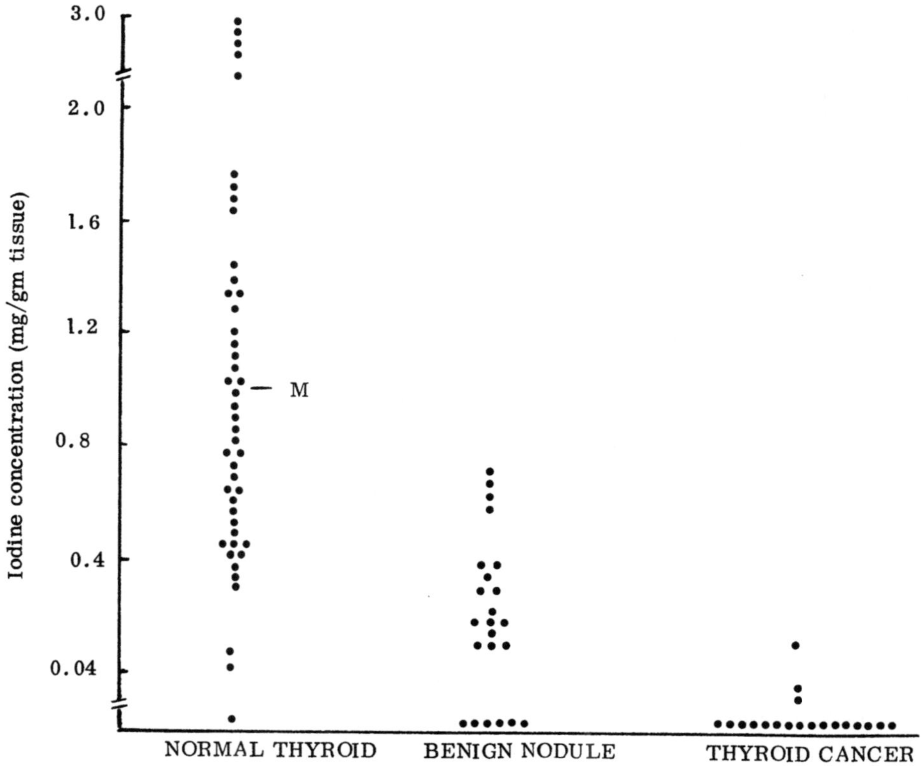

Fig. 4. Stable iodine content of thyroid nodules measured by fluorescent excitation analysis. *M* mean value (Trados 1978)

pointers to malignancy in a thyroid nodule, however, and it is also helpful to bear in mind factors that tend to increase the overall probability of malignancy, such as prior head and neck irradiation, age under 40 in male patients, fixation, hoarseness, lymphadenopathy, fast rate of growth, family history of MCT (GRAZE et al. 1978), and possibly, as recently shown by LIVADAS et al. (1976), the association of a solitary cold nodule with Graves' disease. A number of other methods, usually involving radionuclide imaging of the thyroid, have been investigated as means of further refinement of the basic investigation of the cold nodule; these are shown in Table 3.

None has proved to be sufficiently discriminating to have been adopted as a routine measure, largely due to the poor specificity (methods 1, 2, 3, 4, 7, 8) and the high false-negative rate and interpretation problems with biopsy measurement of the total iodine content of thyroid nodules by quantitative fluorescent excitation analysis is rather more encouraging (PATTON et al. 1976), almost 100% of thyroid malignancies having an undetectable or very low stable iodine content, whereas at least 50% of benign nodules have higher levels (Fig. 4). Thus it may be a technique with a low false-negative rate but a high false-positive rate, which gives a potential for decreasing the number of unnecessary thyroid operations without missing any malignant lesions.

Previously Irradiated Patients

It is now well accepted that irradiation of the head, neck, or upper chest may result in the subsequent development of thyroid cancer, albeit with a long latent period (ARNOLD et al. 1975). A screening programme based on optimal radionuclide imaging techniques will detect more than 95% of the malignant nodules and is markedly more sensitive than clinical examination (ARNOLD et al. 1975). The current status of such screening programs has been summarized by the National Cancer Institute (1976).

Follow-up of Patients with Differentiated Thyroid Malignancies

As with any other malignant tumours that metastasize, routine radionuclide investigations, i.e., bone, brain, or liver scans, etc., may be required for the proper assessment and management of patients with differentiated thyroid malignancies. However, for the purpose of this presentation we shall confine the discussion to specific methods for the follow-up of patients with differentiated functioning thyroid cancer.

In these patients postoperative follow-up investigations have two functions:

1) To assess the completeness of initial surgical or radioiodine ablation of the thyroid and detect residual or recurrent tumour,
2) to assess the probability that there is sufficient uptake of radioiodine by residual tumour to make radioiodine therapy worthwhile.

Currently the most widely used and accepted method of follow-up is regular total-body scanning with radioiodine (^{131}I). The principle of this technique is based on the fact that although differentiated thyroid cancers show little or no iodine uptake in the presence of normal thyroid tissue, following ablation of normal thyroid tissue and in the presence of high blood TSH levels, iodine uptake will take place into residual or metastatic tumour, which can thus be detected as hot lesions on a whole-body scan. This method has three important advantages over other techniques:

1) Sensitive detection of residual tumour in the neck or in distant metastases,
2) spatial localization of the metastases,
3) assessment of potential for radioiodine treatment.

Technique

The patient does not resume thyroid replacement therapy postoperatively, or discontinues thyroid replacement therapy prior to scanning. It is usual to stop thyroxine (T_4) for 4 weeks and triiodothyronine (T_3) for 2 weeks prior to scanning with ^{131}I. In view of the biological half-life of T_4 vs T_3, there is probably not a great deal of difference between these two regimes. What is important, however, both for detection and for treatment, is the level of endogenous TSH stimulation achieved. EDMONDS et al. (1977) have shown the importance of getting the TSH level above 30 mU/litre for adequate uptake into tumour. There is a small proportion of patients, particularly after long-term follow-up, who in spite of apparent complete ablation of the thyroid fail to achieve an adequate TSH level after thyroxine withdrawal (EDMONDS et al. 1977; STAHL and SHAPIRO 1973). Whether this is due to surreptitious self-administration of thyroxine or a truly nonresponsive hypothalamic-pituitary axis is not entirely clear. Between 1 and 15 mCi of ^{131}I is administered orally, after establishing that women patients are not pregnant. The optimal time for the scan is 72 h after the dose of radioiodine (BEKERMAN et al. 1974), when the physiological sites of uptake or secretion (saliva, stomach, kidneys, bladder, colon) have diminished and there is low background activity. The scan is performed with either a rectilinear scanner (ideally with a whole-body attachment) or a gamma camera with multiple views or in a scanning mode. Quantitation may be important in assessment of the subsequent radioiodine dosimetry (THOMAS et al. 1977).

Various adjunctive methods to improve uptake and hence visualization of tumour have been used:

1) Injections of bovine TSH, which are unnecessary when an adequate endogenous TSH level is achieved and may have severe allergic complications (HERSHMAN and EDWARDS 1972; KRISHNAMURTHY 1978),
2) diuretic therapy (HAMBURGER 1969),
3) low-iodine diet to decrease the dilution of radioactive iodine entering the tumour with stable iodine in the plasma (HAMBURGER 1969),
4) antithyroid drugs, taking advantage of the rebound increased uptake shortly after they are discontinued and also the possible blocking of thyroid hormone production by tumour,
5) administration of TRH, which may conceivably be of use in those patients who fail to achieve a good TSH response to thyroxine withdrawal but has not been adequately investigated.

With the possible exceptions of diuretic therapy and low-iodine diet, these methods probably do not increase the sensitivity of the method significantly, and there are no well-controlled studies to support their routine use for the detection of tumour.

Occasionally, whole-body scanning following therapeutic doses of radioiodine (50 mCi and above) may demonstrate lesions not shown by the tracer scan (PREISMAN and HALPER 1978), but it is probably not justifiable as a routine measure because of the technical problems associated with having such a patient in a nuclear medicine department.

Clinical Examples

Case 1. Figure 5a shows a solitary cold thyroid nodule, which on biopsy was shown to be a follicular thyroid carcinoma. Four days after total thyroidectomy no functioning thyroid tissue was demonstrated (Fig. 5b). Four weeks later, without any thyroxine replacement, endogenous serum TSH was > 40 mU/litre and uptake into residual tumour was shown at the site of the primary lesion (Fig. 5c). This case demonstrates the relative lack of uptake of a differentiated tumour in the presence of normal thyroid tissue of normal serum TSH after thyroid ablation, but good tumour uptake of iodine in the presence of high TSH levels. The

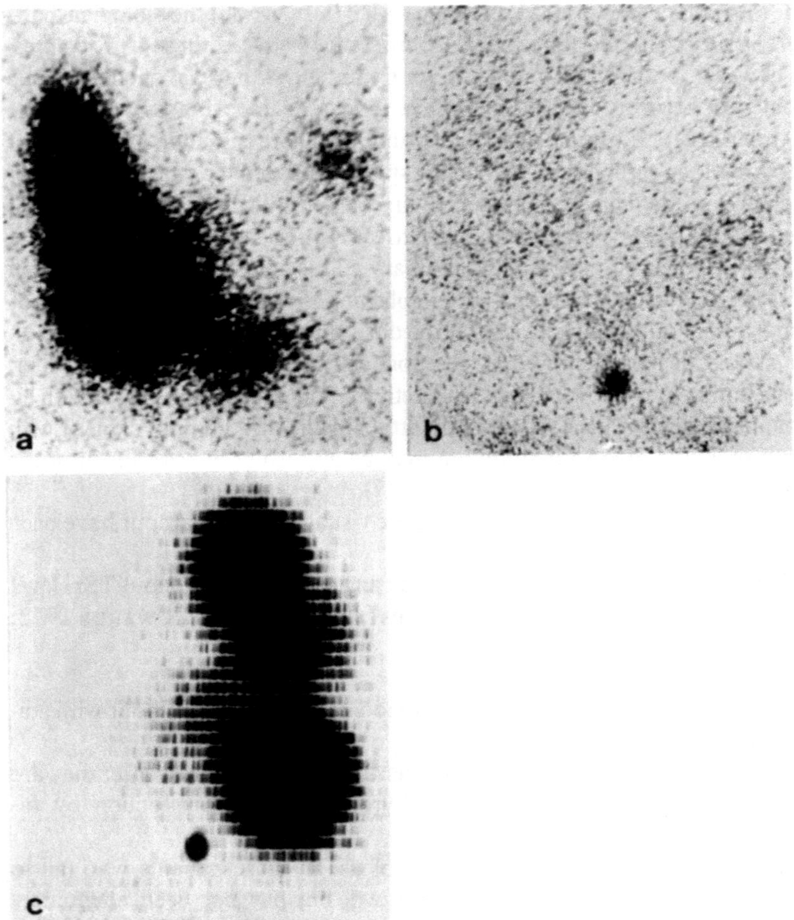

Fig. 5a–c. Follicular thyroid carcinoma. **a** Initial scan; **b** 4 days after total thyroidectomy; **c** 4 weeks after thyroidectomy (residual tumour)

same patient was shown to have extensive metastatic tumour uptake over both lung fields (Fig. 6), while the chest X-ray was initially considered to be normal, confirming the superior sensitivity of radioiodine scan over radiology in detecting functioning pulmonary metastases.

Case 2. The commoner finding after partial or "total" thyroidectomy is illustrated in Fig. 7. The initial scan (Fig. 7a) shows a solitary cold nodule caused by a papillary carcinoma. Immediately after subtotal thyroidectomy, residual normal thyroid tissue in the right love is demonstrated (Fig. 7b). No uptake is seen in the tumour bed. Two months after ablation of the residual normal tissue with 80 mCi ^{131}I, uptake in residual tumour at the original site is demonstrated (Fig. 7c).

Case 3. A whole-body scan after "total" thyroid ablation showed residual tumour uptake in the neck (Fig. 8a), which responded to radioiodine treatment leaving a normal whole-body scan (Fig. 8b).

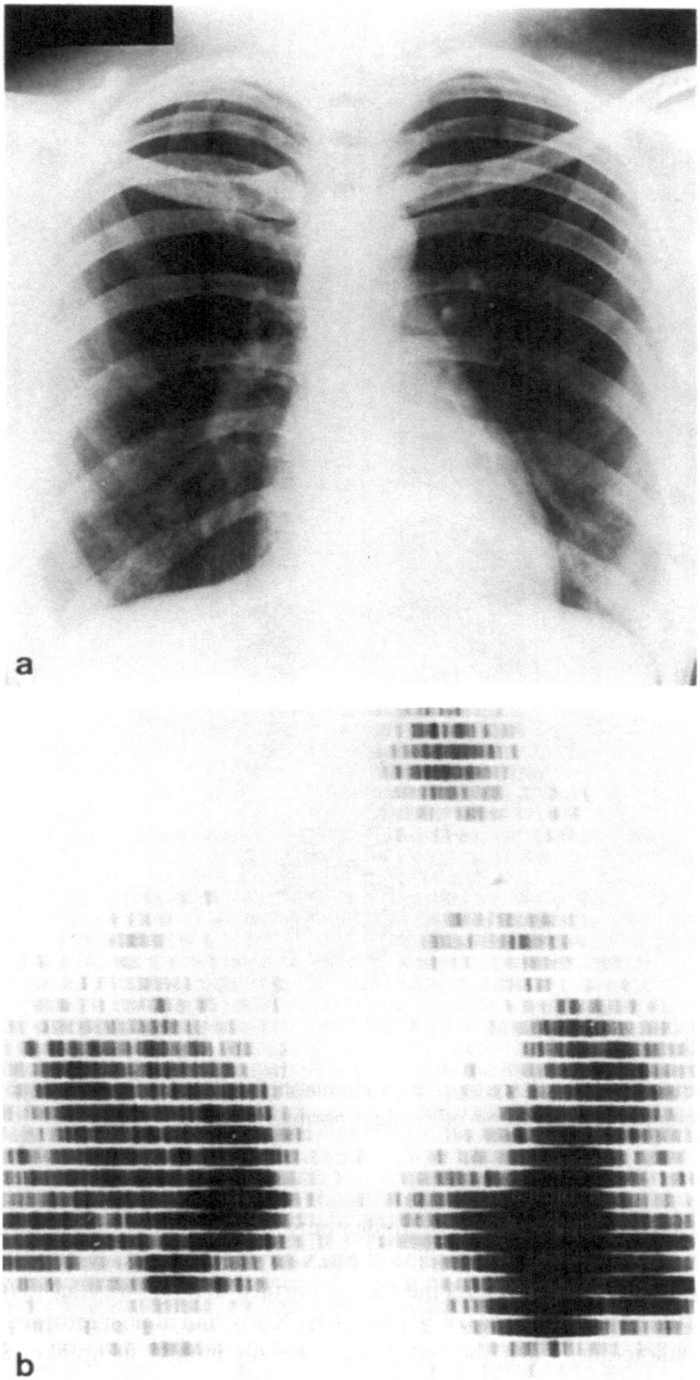

Fig. 6a, b. Functioning thyroid metastases in the lungs after total thyroidectomy. **a** Chest X-ray; **b** ^{131}I scan

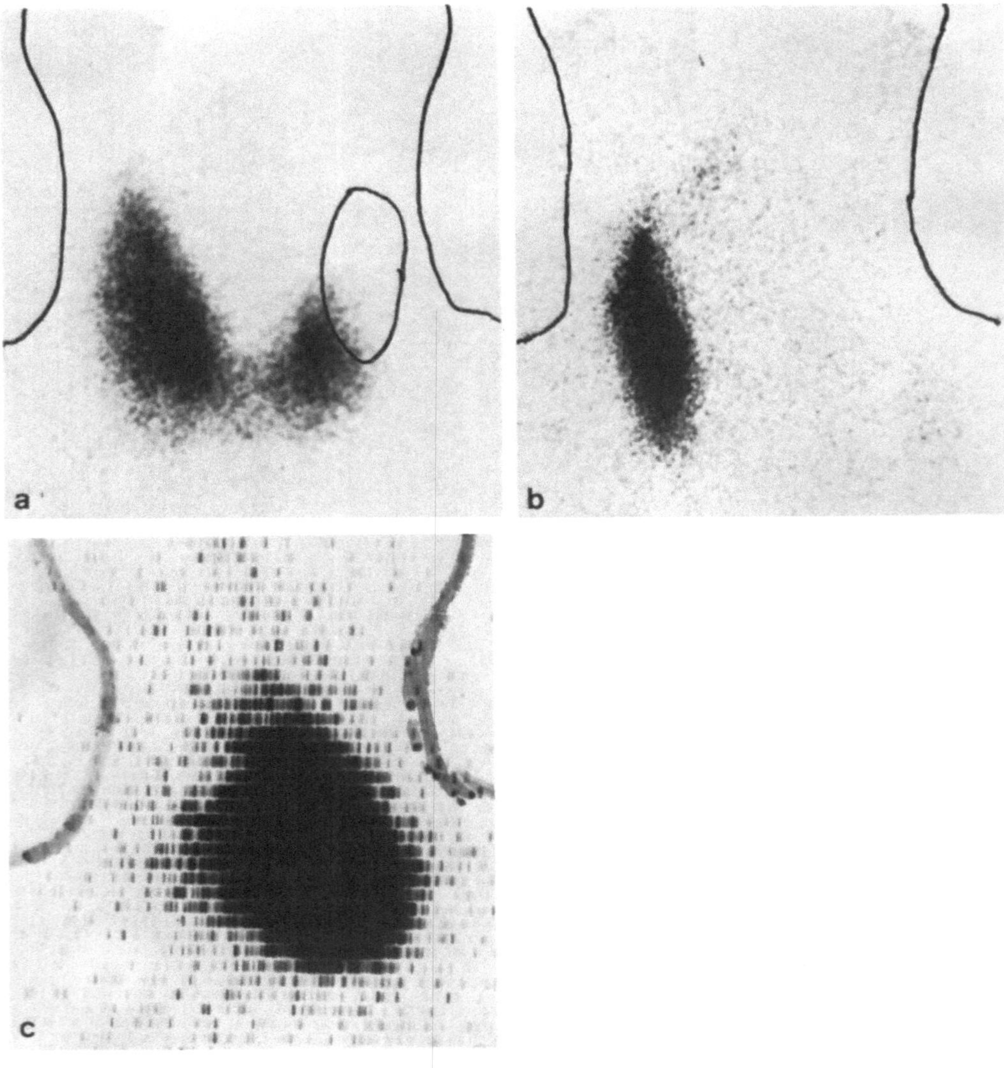

Fig. 7a–c. Papillary thyroid carcinoma before (**a**), 10 days after subtotal thyroidectomy (**b**) and 2 months after ablation of residual normal tissue (**c**)

Case 4. Following total thyroidectomy for a follicular thyroid carcinoma, annual chest X-ray was used for follow-up. The chest X-ray became clearly abnormal after 5 years, follow-up (Fig. 9a), and a radioiodine scan confirmed that this was due to functioning metastases (Fig. 10a). After two doses of ^{131}I the chest X-ray had almost returned to normal (Fig. 9b) and the radioiodine scans showed progressive diminution in uptake (Fig. 10b and c).

Case 5. A poorly differentiated follicular thyroid carcinoma was exposed initially to successful radioiodine therapy but the patient later presented with a haemoptysis. A chest X-ray (Fig. 11a) showed a mass at the right base and the left hilum; a radioiodine scan (Fig. 11b) showed that the right-sided lesion took up tracer well but the one on the left did not. The pa-

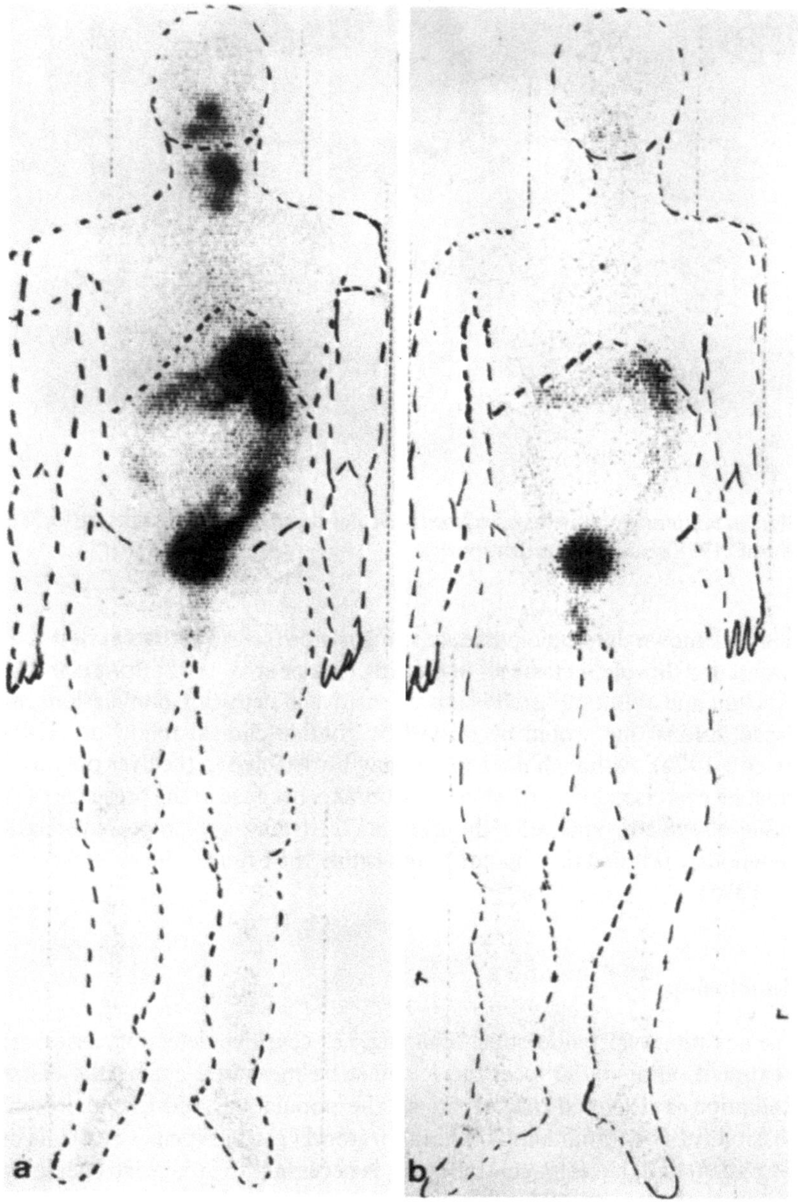

Fig. 8a, b. Differentiated thyroid tumour before (**a**) and after (**b**) ^{131}I therapy (^{131}I whole-body scan)

tient refused further treatment and died shortly after. At autopsy the right lesion was found to contain relatively well-differentiated thyroid carcinoma but the left lesion consisted almost entirely of anaplastic cells. This shows that metastases do not always concentrate iodine, depending on the degree of differentiation, and therefore may not respond to radioiodine treatment in the same way as well-differentiated tumours.

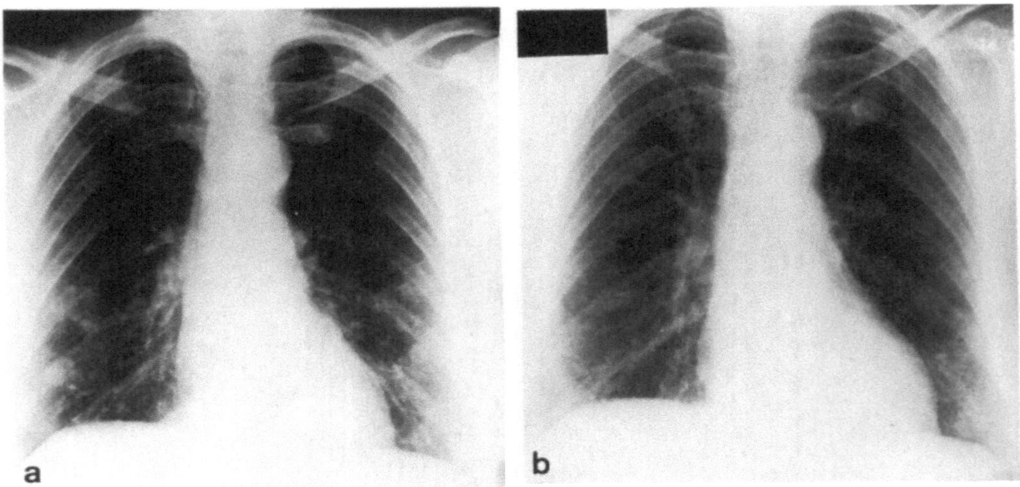

Fig. 9a, b. Pulmonary metastases from follicular thyroid carcinoma before (**a**, May 1977) and after (**b**, March 1978) radioiodine therapy

It is well known that radioiodine scanning is more sensitive than a chest X-ray in detecting differentiated thyroid metastases in the lung (Henk et al. 1972; Bonte and McConnell 1973; Turner and Weir 1972). It is more sensitive in detecting bony lesions, and will detect soft-tissue lesions that would be missed by routine clinical follow-up (Krishnamurthy and Blahd 1972). Although metastases may be detected in the liver only by ^{131}I scanning, care must be exercised in interpreting liver uptake, because in the presence of functioning thyroid tissue elsewhere, uptake in the liver at 72 h may only represent degradation of the endogenously labelled thyroid hormones rather than functioning metastases (Woolfender et al. 1975).

Conclusions

The advantages of radioiodine scanning, i.e., sensitive detection, assessment for radioiodine treatment, and spatial localization, must be measured against its disadvantages, i.e.: (1) Radiation is delivered the to patient, the population, and the environment; (2) there is a possibility of contamination of the laboratory; (3) it is expensive; (4) it is time-consuming for the patient and the technical staff; (5) it is necessary to induce iatrogenic hypothyroidism; (6) a recurrent rise in TSH may stimulate the growth of the tumour.

These disadvantages are especially important if, as in many centres, the practice is to scan at regular, e.g., 6-monthly, intervals until the scan is negative.

Other methods that can be used as an alternative or in addition are:

1) Profile scanning (Pochin 1971), which is sensitive but is associated with relatively poor spatial resolution, which makes the likelihood of missing lesions near physiological sites of uptake high,
2) measurement of serum PB ^{131}I, usually at 72 h or 5 days, which is a sensitive method but lacks spatial resolution. It may be used in conjunction with total-body scanning or profile scanning (Pochin 1971),

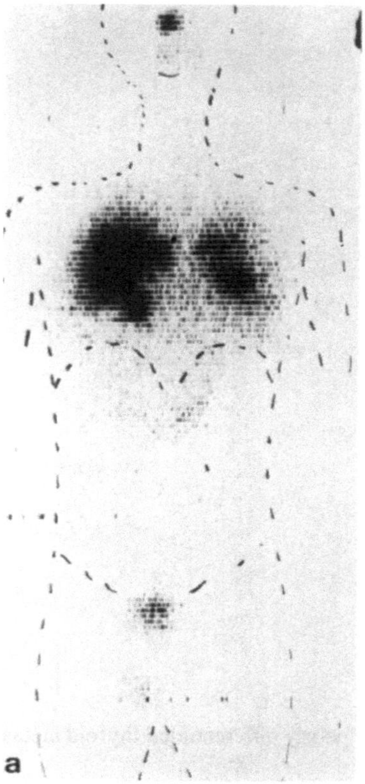

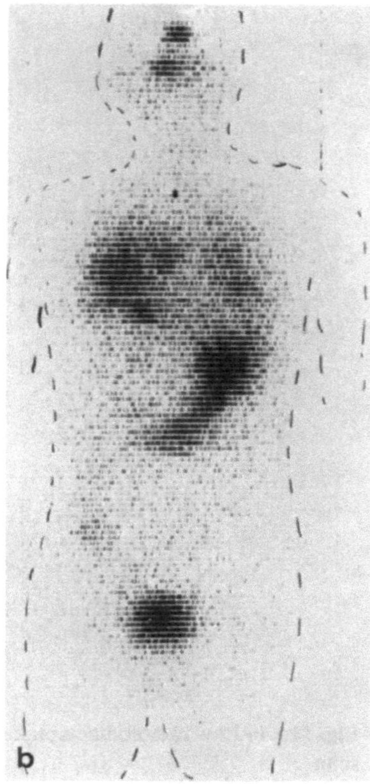

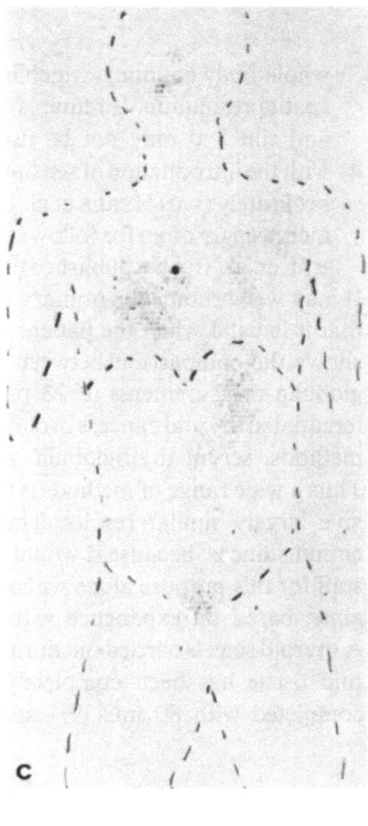

Fig. 10a–c. Whole-body radioiodine scan corresponding to chest X-rays in Fig. 9. **a** May 1977; **b** August 1977; **c** March 1978

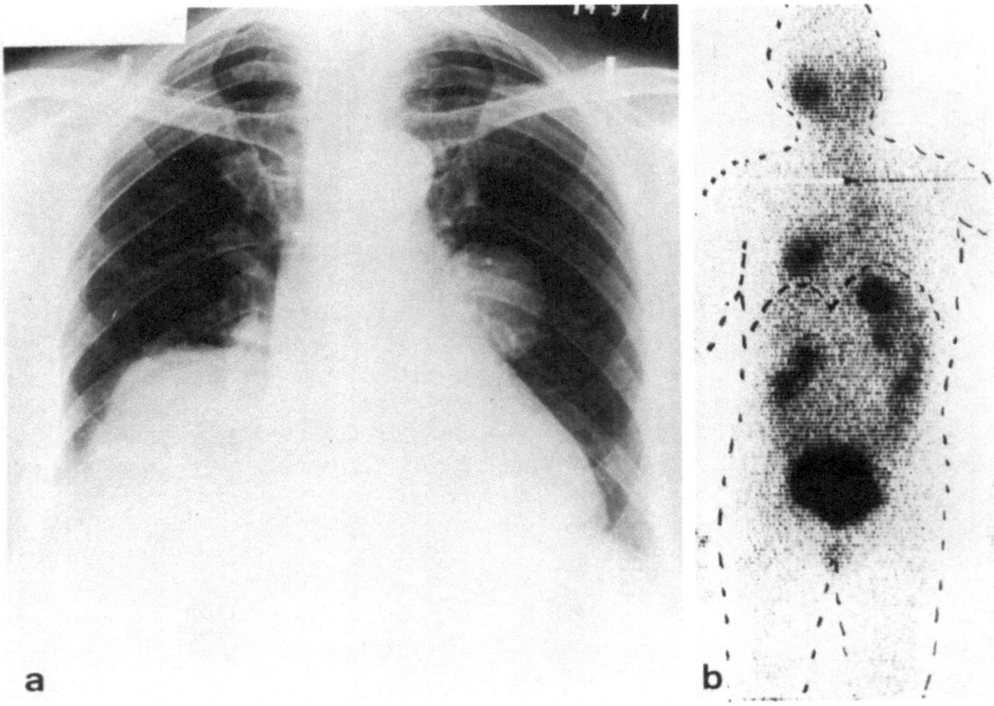

Fig. 11a, b. Low radioiodine uptake by poorly differentiated thyroid metastases. **a** chest X-ray; **b** ^{131}I scan

3) whole-body counting, which is also a sensitive and quantitative technique but again lacks spatial resolution. It requires access to a whole-body counter, which is expensive to buy and run and may not be used to capacity (EDMONDS et al. 1970),
4) with the introduction of sensitive radioimmunoassay methods for measuring thyroglobulin accurately (VAN HERLE et al. 1973), serial serum thyroglobulin measurement is being used increasingly often for follow-up [VAN HERLE et al. 1973; LO GERFO et al. 1977; NG TANG FUI et al. (to be published)].

It may well become the primary method of choice in the future, especially if it can be shown that it is valid when the patient is receiving full suppressive doses of thyroxine. Figure 12 shows the comparison between whole-body iodine scans and simultaneous serum thyroglobulin measurements in 23 patients who had undergone total thyroid ablation for differentiated thyroid cancers in our institution. There is an excellent correlation between the two methods, serum thyroglobulin measurement possibly being the more sensitive.

Thus a wide range of methods is currently available, and if used carefully these will probably give largely similar results. The particular choice will depend to some extent on local circumstances, because it would be uneconomical to obtain expensive equipment and train staff for this purpose alone without reference to other potential uses. At present our own regime, based on experience with 42 patients over the last 5 years, is as follows:

A thyroid scan is carried out during the first postoperative week to assess whether normal thyroid tissue has been completely or partially ablated. If incomplete, thyroid ablation is completed with 80 mCi ^{131}I and thyroid replacement is given for 2 months.

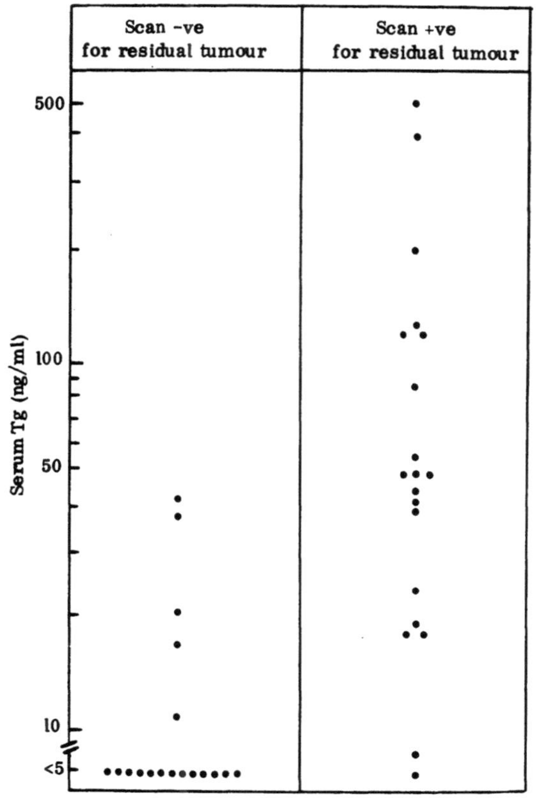

Fig. 12. Serum Tg level and whole-body radioiodine scan in 23 patients following total thyroid ablation for differentiated carcinoma

Table 4. Follow-up scintigraphy in 42 patients[a] with differentiated thyroid cancer[b]

Time of scan	No. of patients	
1st week postop.		Scan + ve
Total thyroidectomy	13	5
STT, lobectomy, biopsy	29	15 (14 not scanned)
6 weeks after ablation	35	24
> 6 months after ablation	27	12

[a] Patients were aged 20–80 years and the follow-up period was > 6 months to > 5 years. Two patients died

[b] Histological examination revealed papillary carcinoma in 31 cases, follicular carcinoma in ten, and follicular and anaplastic in one

Three months after ablation by radioiodine and partial thyroidectomy, *or* 6 weeks after total ablation by surgery alone without any intervening thyroid replacement, a whole-body scan is performed to assess residual or metastatic tumour uptake. If any is demonstrated, the patient is treated with 150 mCi ^{131}I. The scan, and further ^{131}I therapy if necessary, are repeated at 6-monthly intervals until abnormal uptake is no longer seen. Suppressive doses of thyroxine are given except for 1 month before each scan.
The whole-body scan is then carried out annually until it remains clear for 2 consecutive years. There is some evidence, however, that when metastases are present initially, the follow-up should be continued for as long as 10–20 years (Krishnamurthy and Blahd 1972; Gardet et al 1978). Table 4 summarizes the findings in 42 patients investigated and treated at Guy's Hospital.

Acknowledgements. S. Ng Tang Fui is supported by a research grant from the Special Trustees of Guy's Hospital. We are indebted to Professor Hoffenberg and Miss E. Black for the thyroglobulin measurements, and to Dr. B. King for the ultrasound scans. We are grateful to Miss H. Upperton for typing the manuscript, and to the Nuclear Medicine technicians for consistently producing high-quality images.

References

1 Alderson PO, Sumner HW, Siegel BA (1976) The single palpable thyroid nodule. Cancer 37:258–265
2 Arnold J, Pinsky, S, Ryo UY, Frohman L, Schneider A, Favus M, Stachura M, Arnold M, Colman M (1975) ^{99m}Tc Pertechnetate thyroid scintigraphy in patients predisposed to thyroid neoplasm by prior radiotherapy to the head and neck. Radiology 115:653–657
3 Beierwaltes WH (1978) The treatment of thyroid carcinoma with radioactive iodine. Semin Nucl Med 8:79–94
4 Bekerman C, Gottschalk A, Hoffer PB (1974) Optimal time for ^{131}I total body imaging to detect metastatic thyroid carcinoma. J Nucl Med Allied Sci 15:477
5 Bonte FJ, McConnell RW (1973) Pulmonary metastases from differentiated thyroid carcinoma demonstrable only by nuclear imaging. Radiology 107:585–590
6 Cowan RJ (1976) Thyroid imaging with radionuclides. South-eastern chapter, Society of nuclear medicine, Atlanta Georgia, continuing education lectures. A review of nuclear medicine, part I, pp 2.1–2.15
7 Edmonds CJ, Smith T, Barnaby CF (1970) Follow-up of thyroid carcinoma by whole body counting. Br J Radiol 43:868–875
8 Edmonds CJ, Hyes S, Kermode JC, Thompson BD (1977) Measurement of serum TSH and thyroid hormones in the management of treatment of thyroid cyarcinoma with radioiodine. Br J Radiol 50:799–807
9 Fukuchi M, Tachibana K, Kuwata K, Nishikawa A, Hyodo K, Okamoto E, Nagai K (1978) Thallium-201 imaging in a thyroid carcinoma – Appearance of a lymph node metastasis. J Nucl Med Allied Sci 19:195–196
10 Galvan G (1977) Thin needle aspiration biopsy and cytological examination of hypofunctional 'cold' thyroid nodules in routine clinical work. Clin Nucl Med 2:413–421
11 Gardet P, Parmentier C, Gerard-Marchant R, L'heritier C, Caillou B, Cukersztein W, Tubiana M (1977) Differentiated cancers of the thyroid: Course after treatment with special reference to frequency and chronology of the first relapse for 470 treated patients. Ann Radiol (Paris) 20:831–840

12 Goolden AWG, Glass BA, Silvester DJ (1968) The choice of a radioactive isotope for the investigation of thyroid disorders. Br J Radiol 41:20–25
13 Graze K, Spiler IJ, Tashjian AH, Melvin KEW, Cevvi-Skinner G, Gagel RF, Miller HH, Wolfe HJ, De Lellis RA, Leape L, Feldman ZT, Reichlin S (1978) Natural history of familial medullary thyroid carcinoma. Effect of a program for early diagnosis. N Engl J Med 299:980–985
14 Hamburger JI (1969) Diuretic augmentation of ^{131}I uptake in inoperable thyroid cancer. N Engl J Med 280:1091–1094
15 Henk JM, Kirkman S, Owen GM (1972) Whole body scanning and ^{131}I therapy in the management of thyroid carcinoma. Br J Radiol 45:369–376
16 Hershman JM, Edwards CL (1972) Serum Thyrotropin (TSH) levels after thyroid ablation compared with TSH levels after exogenous bovine TSH; Implications for ^{131}I treatment of thyroid carcinoma. J Clin Endocrinol Metab 34:814–818
17 Hurley PJ, Strauss HW, Pavoni P, Langan JK, Wagner HN Jr (1971) The scintillation camera with pinhole collimator in thyroid imaging. Radiology 101:133
18 Kaplan WD, Holman BL, Selenkow HA, Davis MA, Holmes RA, Isitman AT, Chandler HL (1974) ^{67}Ga-Citrate and the non-functioning thyroid nodule. J Nucl Med Allied Sci 15:424–427
19 Karelitz JR, Richards JB (1975) Necessity of oblique views in evaluating the functional status of a thyroid nodule. J Nucl Med Allied Sci 15:782–785
20 Koutras DA, Pandos PG, Sfontouris J, Koukoulomati-Speritza A, Psarras A, Malamos (1976) Thyroid scanning with Gallium-67 and Cesium-131. J Nucl Med Allied Sci 17:268–271
21 Kristhnamurthy GT (1978) Human reaction to bovine TSH. J Nucl Med Allied Sci 19:284–286
22 Krishnamurthy GT, Blahd WH (1972) Diagnostic and therapeutic implications of long term radioisotope scanning in the management of thyroid cancer. J Nucl Med Allied Sci 13:924–927
23 Lahey FH (1953) Preoperative diagnosis of carcinoma of the thyroid in surgery of the thyroid. Surg Clin North Am 33:781–792
24 Livadas D, Psarras A, Koutras DA (1976) Malignant cold thyroid nodules in hyperthyroidism. Br J Surg 63:726–728
25 Lo Gerfo P, Stillman T, Colacchio D, Feind C (1977) Serum Thyroglobulin and recurrent thyroid cancer. Lancet 1:881–882
26 Ma M, Ong GB (1975) Cystic thyroid nodules. Br J Surg 62:205
27 Maisey MN, Moses DC, Hurley PJ, Wagner HN Jr (1963) Improved methods for thyroid scanning. JAMA 223:761–763
28 Massin JP, Plauchon C, Perez R (1977) Comparison of ^{99m}Tc-Pertechnetate and ^{131}I in scanning of thyroid nodules. Clin Nucl Med 2:324–333
29 Meybier H, Claussen C, Nievergelt J, Wahl R (1978) Computerised tomography in retrosternal goitre and cold thyroid nodules. Abstract of the 9th annual meeting of the European Thyroid Association, Berlin. Ann Endocrinol (Paris) 39:(5) A 18
30 Miskin M, Rosen IB, Walfish PG (1973) B-mode ultrasonography in the assessment of thyroid gland lesions. Ann Intern Med 79:505–510
31 National Cancer Institute (1976) U.S. Department of health, education and welfare: Irradiation-related thyroid cancer. Information for Physicians. DHEW Publication No (NIH) 77–1120, Washington
32 Ng Tang Fui S, Maisey MN (to be published) Radionuclide thyroid scanning. Hospital Update
33 Patton JA, Hollifield JN, Brill AB, Lee GS, Patton DD (1976) Differentiation between malignant and benign solitary thyroid nodules by fluorescent scanning. J Nucl Med Allied Sci 17:17–21
34 Perlmutter M, Slater SL (1956) Which nodular goitres should be removed? N Engl J Med 255:65–71

35 Pochin EE (1971) Radioiodine therapy of thyroid cancer. Semin Nucl Med 1:503–515
36 Preisman RA, Halpern S (1978) Detection of metastatic thyroid carcinoma after the administration of a therapeutic dose of ^{131}I-Iodine. Eur J Nucl Med 3:69–70
37 Psarras A, Papadopoulos SN, Livadas D, Pharmakiolis AD, Koutras DA (1972) The single thyroid nodule. Br J Surg 59:545–548
38 Ryo UY, Arnold J, Colman M, Arnold M, Favus M, Frohman L, Schneider A, Stachura M, Pinsky S (1976) Thyroid scintigram. Sensitivity with Sodium Pertechnetate Tc^{99m} and gamma camera with pinhole collimator. JAMA 235:1235–1238
39 Stahl TJ, Shapiro B (1973) Use of human thyrotropin radioimmunoassay in management of patients with thyroid carcinoma. J Nucl Med Allied Sci 14:900–902
40 Tadros TG (1978) Fluorescent excitation analysis in clinical and endocrinological investigations. Ph. D. dissertation University of London
41 Thomas SR, Maxon HR, Kereiakes JG, Saenger EL (1977) Quantitative external counting techniques enabling improved diagnostic and therapeutic decisions in patients with well differentiated thyroid cancer. Radiology 122:731–737
42 Turner JE, Weir GJ (1972) Pulmonary metastases from thyroid carcinoma detectable only by ^{131}I scan. Treatment and response. J Nucl Med Allied Sci 13:852–855
43 Herle AJ van, Uller RP, Matthews NL, Brown J (1973) Radioimmunoassay for measurement of thyroglobulin in human serum. J Clin Invest 52:1320–1327
44 Herle AJ van, Uller RP (1975) Elevated serum thyroglobulin. A marker for metastases in differentiated thyroid carcinoma. J Clin Invest 56:272–277
45 Wang CA, Vickery AL, Maloof F (1976) The role of needle biopsy in evaluating solitary cold thyroid nodules. In: Robbins J, Braverman L (eds) Thyroid research. Proceedings of the seventh International Thyroid Conference. Excerpta Medica, Amsterdam Oxford, American Elsevier, New York, pp 568–570
46 Weinstein MB, Ashkar FS, Caron CD (1971) ^{75}Se Selenomethionine as a scanning agent for the differential diagnosis of the cold thyroid nodule. Semin Nucl Med 1:390–396
47 Wellman HN, Anger RT Jr (1971) Radioiodine dosimetry and the use of radioiodines other than ^{131}I in thyroid diagnosis. Semin Nucl Med 1:356–378
48 Wolfstein RS (1978) Enigma of the hyperfunctioning thyroid carcinoma resolved. J Nucl Med Allied Sci 19:441–442
49 Woolfender JM, Waxman AD, Wolfstein RS, Siemsen JK (1975) Scintigraphic evaluation of liver metastases from thyroid carcinoma. J Nucl Med 16:669–671

Radiological Assessment

B. Eddleston

Christie Hospital and Holt Radium Insitute, GB-Manchester, M20 9BX

Introduction

The thyroid gland is a readily accessible structure – accessible to the clinician's vision, his palpating fingers, the exploratory needle, and the surgeon's scalpel.
Radiological assessment of thyroid cancer is determined by this accessibility, the mode of presentation of the primary lesion, distant spread of disease, the possibility of associated abnormalities in other structures and, in survivors, the complications of management.

Ultrasonography

In recent years there has been considerable emphasis on the role of ultrasonic scanning in the evaluation of the solitary thyroid nodule found to be "cold" on ^{131}I tracer testing. The ratio of malignant to benign nodules is higher in younger age groups. Many so-called single nodules are part of a multinodular goitre, with an incidence as high as 50% in some series (Vander et al. 1968). Messaris et al. (1973) reported a 10% incidence of malignancy in cold nodules. Taylor (1958) quoted figures of up to 25%, and there have been other series with incidences of over 40%.
The majority of reports on ultrasonic scanning have been concerned with the differentiation of cysts from solid lesions.
Blum et al. (1972) claimed an accurate correlation between thyroid sonography and surgical removal in 13 cysts and 54 solid lesions over 1 cm in diameter, a critical dimension referred to in several other reports. Blum et al. (1973) did not consider sonography to be of value in distinguishing between malignant and benign lesions.
The need for high gain settings during scanning was stressed by Miskin et al. (1973). Cysts showed persistence of sonolucency, the presence of a thin, discrete posterior wall, and echoes only from the anterior wall. Solid lesions revealed interior echoes and no posterior wall definition. Among 50 cases submitted to surgery, ultrasound was accurate in diagnosing 11 cystic and 39 solid lumps.
In the series of 86 cases reported by Thijs (1971), four cases of thyroid carcinoma were not differentiated by ultrasound.
However, Taylor et al. (1974) stated that the high-quality grayscale technique could show up the presence of malignant disease by revealing defects in the regular arrangement of normal glandular tissue.
Hales et al. (1978) have commented further on the characteristics of echo patterns in relation to thyroid nodules. They have defined a picture – well-defined localized area with low-level

echoes – into which most malignant lesions fall, but stress that benign conditions may simulate this appearance and that a clear diagnosis of cancer cannot be made on echo patterns alone.

Thermography

SAMUELS (1972) describing the use of thermography in the assessment of thyroid disease, referred to the value of this technique in differentiating benign and malignant nodules when taken into account together with ^{131}I scanning. In an ambient temperature of 68° F, alcohol was applied to cool the examined area and a hot thermogram associated with a nodule that was cold on radioidine scanning was considered to be indicative of malignant disease.
The majority of cases presenting with thyroid cancer in our clinics, however, do so with an obvious mass in the neck, of varying size. There are exceptions, but they are rare. We have seen only two cases of lingual thyroid cancer in the past 20 year (Fig. 1.) Not infrequently there is a history of the presence of a lump for many years. Some may have been biopsied in the past and reported as benign. A few patients have undergone total or subtotal thyroidectomy because of the size of the lesion and its fixity and consistency or because the patient has become worried about the continued presence of the thyroid swelling.

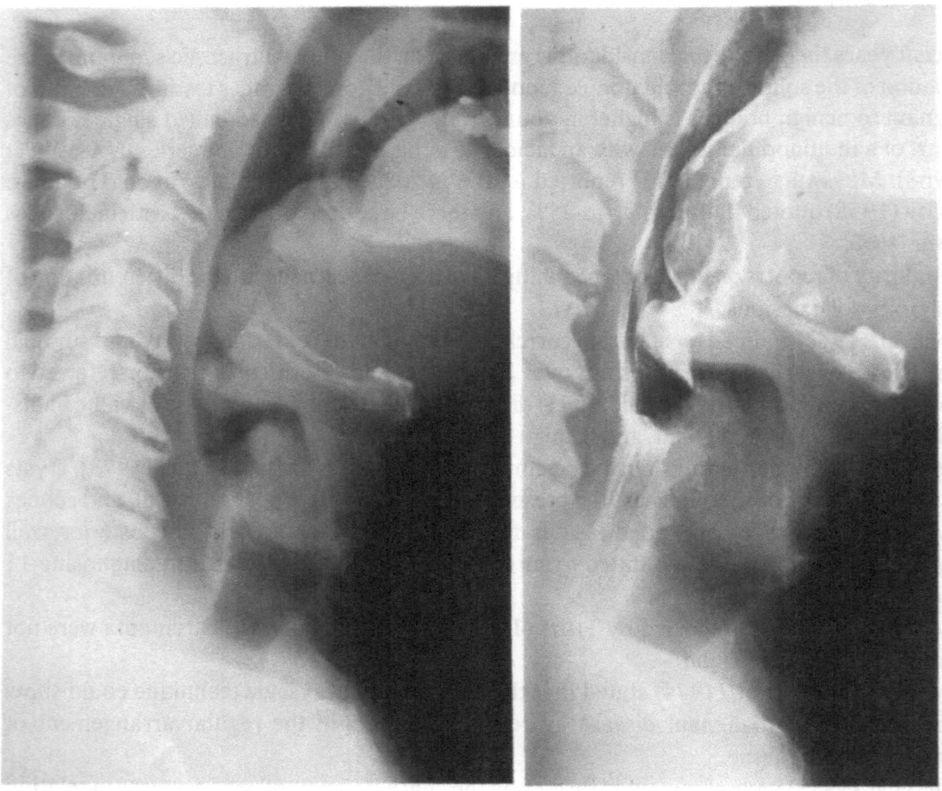

Fig. 1. Large lobulated lingual mass reaching to the vallecula

Radiography

Initial X-ray assessment, in those with a mass lesion, is based on soft-tissue radiography of the neck and thoracic inlet, with the Valsalva manoeuvre, together with chest examination. The chest radiograph defines the extent of the mass with special reference to mediastinal extension, effects on local structures (especially the trachea), presence of calcification (whether in tumour or palpable nodes), and status of hilar/mediastinal lymph node areas and the lung field appearances. Suspicion of direct invasion of the upper airway may require linear or transaxial tomography of the larynx and trachea (Fig. 2). Occasionally a thyroid cancer may present as a posterior mediastinal mass.

The angiographic appearances of thyroid malignancy – abnormal vessel patterns, irregularity and heterogenicity of tumour staining, and ragged contour of the gland – were described by TAKAHASHI et al. (1969), who reported a diagnostic accuracy rate of 90%.

Calcification related to thyroid masses may or may not be a direct index of malignancy. McDONALD (1970) and DEGROOT and STANBURY (1975) have stressed fine stippling in papillary adenocarcinoma.

Large, dense, amorphous plaques or ring shadows are usually regarded as more typical of benign disease, but their presence does not exempt the gland from being affected by carcinoma. A diagnosis of calcified tuberculous nodes enveloped by the tumour should be made with caution. KEISER (1973) reported a 35% incidence of amorphous calcification in the neck in medullary thyroid cancer.

The X-ray views described may be of further value in assessment of the effectiveness of radio- or chemotherapy in reducing the size of the primary tumour and in relieving pressure effects on adjacent structures (Fig. 3). The chest examination also affords an important baseline for future management when related to metastatic disease.

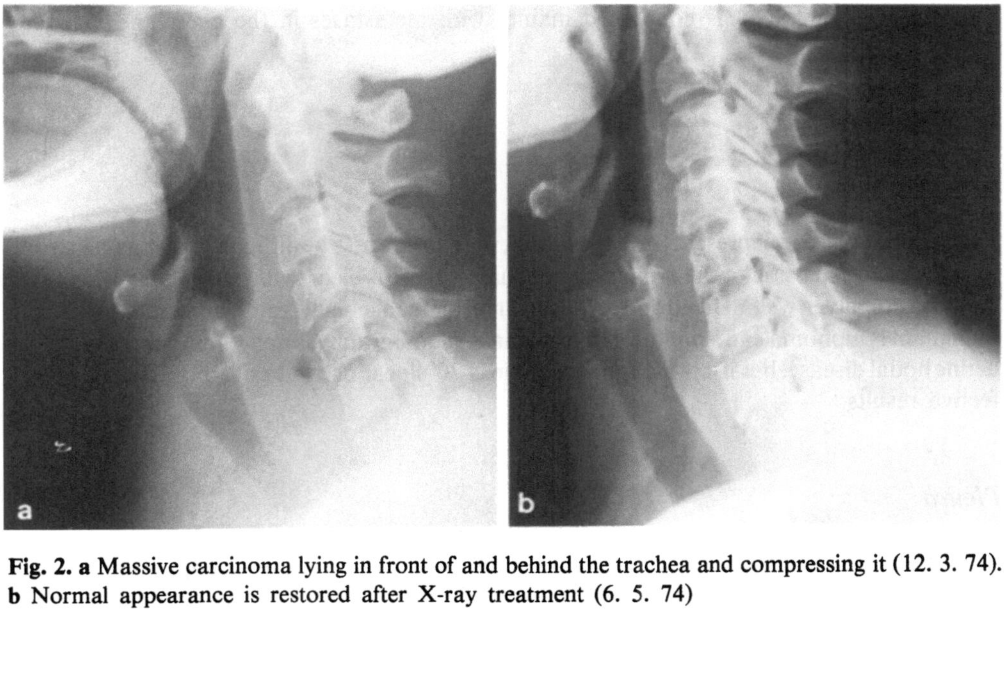

Fig. 2. a Massive carcinoma lying in front of and behind the trachea and compressing it (12. 3. 74). **b** Normal appearance is restored after X-ray treatment (6. 5. 74)

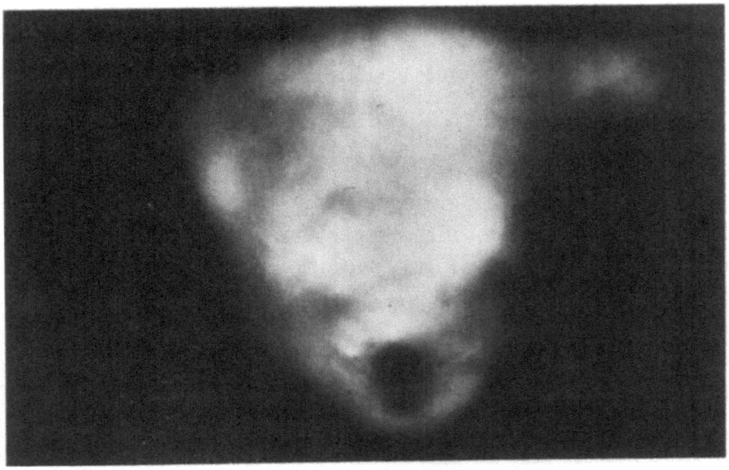

Fig. 3. Transaxial tomogram through the neck, with thyroid mass lying anterior to the trachea

Assessment of Metastatic Disease

An analysis of a group of patients dying of thyroid cancer with metastatic disease (registered at the Christie Hospital and Holt Radium Institute, Manchester) showed the following site distribution.

Lymph nodes (local/regional)	46%
Lung	39%
Bone	33%
Liver	13%
Brain	11%

Conventional radiology is concerned mainly with metastases in the chest and in bone.

Chest

Mediastinum

Lymph node disease, if present from the outset, may sometimes be difficult to distinguish from intrathoracic extension of the primary lesion, unless there is clear evidence of lobulation (Fig. 4). Occasionally, a well-defined and localized anterior mediastinal lymph node enlargement in malignant lymphoma can simulate a thyroid mass. Tomography is not commonly required to define nodal disease, but if it is thought desirable, a 20° linear or transaxial movement gives effective results.

Pleura

Metastases may be associated with a pleural effusion though these do not appear to be so frequent as in breast cancer, for example. Pleural fluid will obscure the deposits and has to be re-

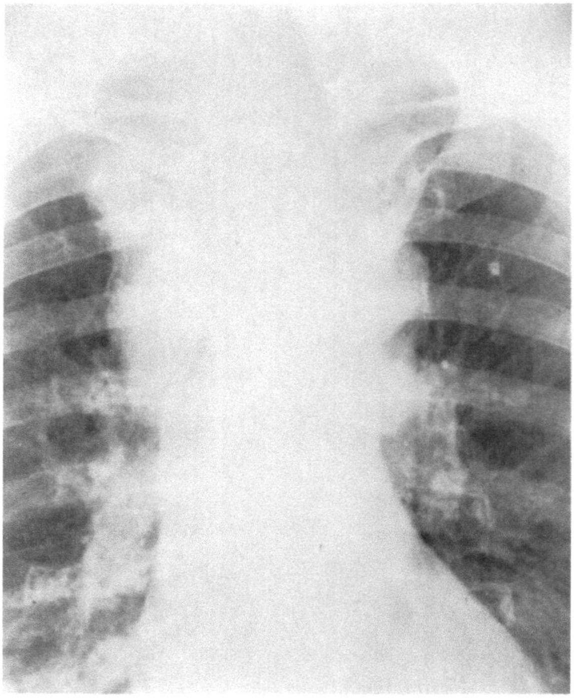

Fig. 4. Mediastinal and paratracheal adenopathy

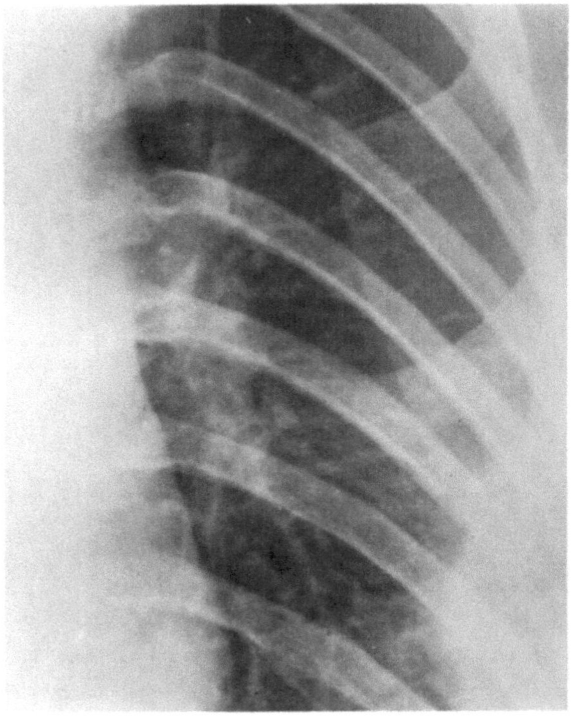

Fig. 5. Pleural metastasis

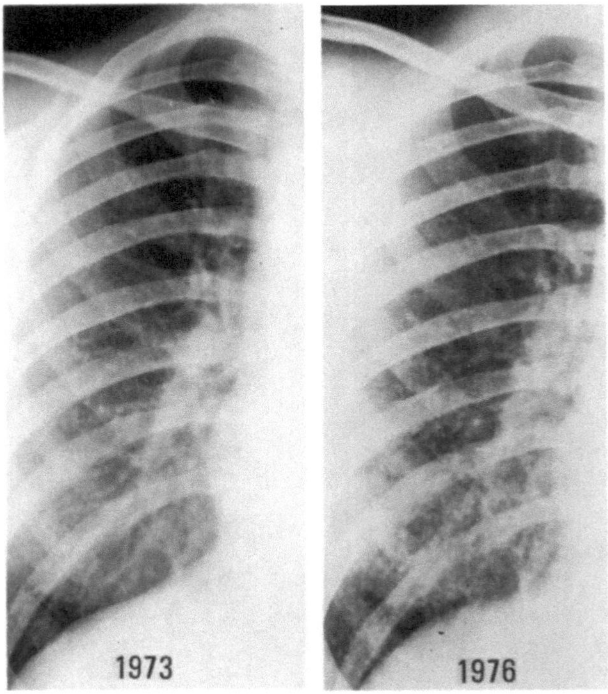

Fig. 6. Lung metastases from papillary adenocarcinoma. Thyroid cancer was not diagnosed until 1976

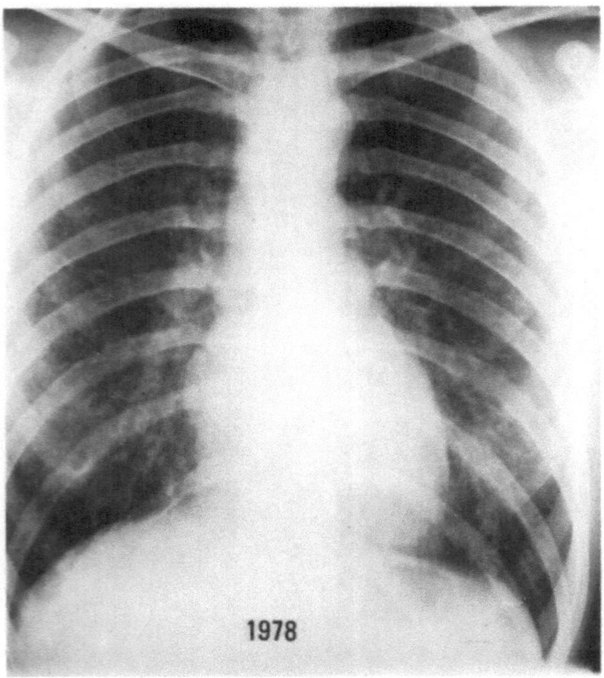

Fig. 7. X-ray plate of same patient as in Fig. 6, taken in 1978 and showing state of resolution after surgery, ^{131}I therapy, and thyroxine medication

moved before X-ray demonstration is possible. Postero-anterior (PA), penetrated antero-posterior (AP), and oblique views may all be necessary to show focal pleural shadows, but care should be taken to eliminate rib metastases as a cause of the pleural opacity (Fig. 5).

Lungs

Three differing patterns of metastases may be seen in the lungs:
1) Discrete, well-defined, cannon-ball shadows varying in size,
2) fine nodular deposits, sometimes miliary in type,
3) coarsening of the bronchovascular striation; a coarse infiltrate (KEISER 1973).

The role of whole-lung tomography has often been stressed in relation to the demonstration of metastases in the lung parenchyma. We have made frequent use of this technique but are not particularly impressed with it in critical appraisal against good-quality baseline and follow-up plain film examination (Figs. 6 and 7).

Bone

Metastases in bone tissue are usually osteolytic in character, and may be very destructive (Fig. 8). Pure sclerotic lesions are rare (SHERMAN et al. 1950) (Fig. 9). There is seldom any periosteal response in the absence of pathological fracture, whose occurrence, as in other me-

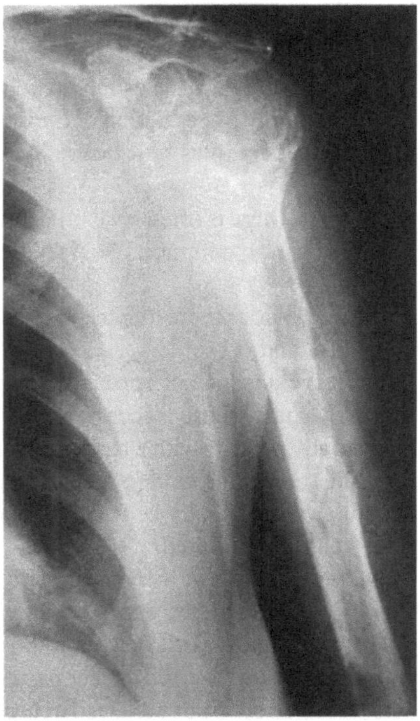

Fig. 8. Extensive destruction in left humerus caused by anaplastic primary tumour

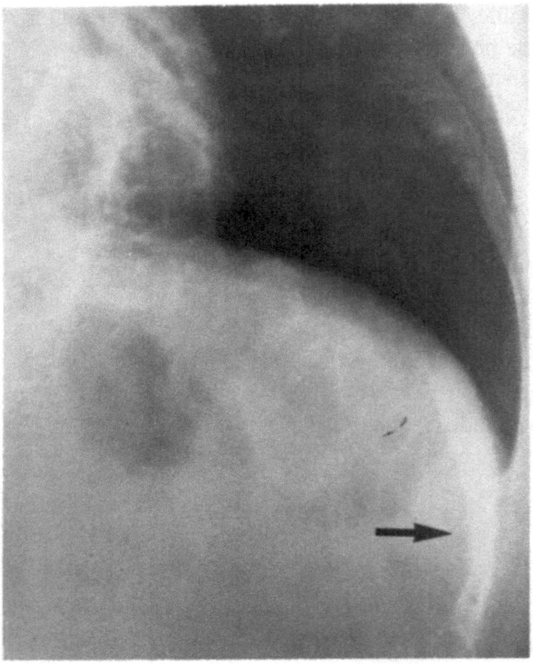

Fig. 9. Sclerotic rib metastasis from medullary carcinoma

tastatic disease, is simply related to the amount of bone mineral removed by the tumour at a particular site. Any area of the skeleton may be involved, but lesions beyond the elbow or the knee are very uncommon, as with other malignancies.

There should be no difficulty in identifying deposits in long bones and the skull. Any problem in the spine and pelvis is usually resolved by linear tomography, stereoscopy, or films in obliquity, or simply by repetition of the doubtful projection after the lapse of a few hours, when intestinal gas shadows will normally have changed sufficiently to confirm or exclude suspicion.

In the spine there is often very little in the way of a paraspinal mass, and major vertebral body collapse is not common. Solitary lesions in this area may sometimes simulate plasmacytoma.

In the iliac blades there may be a multilocular appearance not unlike that of giant-cell tumour. (Figs. 10 and 11).

Even in the absence of specific therapy, metastases may show little progression over some time. After apparently successful treatment there is never good restoration of bone; a lytic defect usually persists with a tendency for the edges to sclerose, and in large areas of involvement lace-like trabeculae tend to form. Metastatic lesions, though showing evidence of this kind of healing, will frequently be found to take up ^{131}I for a considerable time if the primary tumour was well-differentiated.

Metastatic disease in the vertebrae is of special importance, in that paraplegia may develop slowly and, having become fully established, may resolve extremely well after decompression plus local radiation and/or radioiodine therapy. Halnan and Roberts (1967) described nine cases among 700 thyroid cancer patients registered at the Christie Hospital, Manchester, over a 20-year period. Four achieved complete recovery. All nine had radiographic evidence of dis-

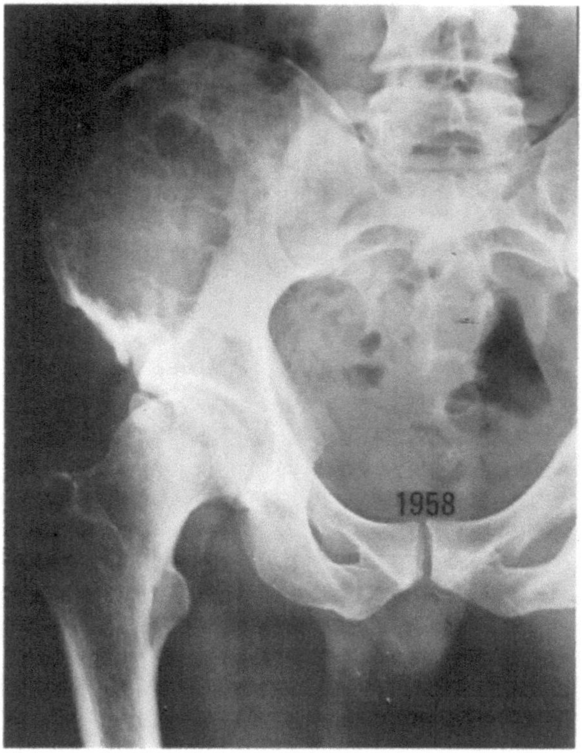

Fig. 10. Ilial metastasis from follicular carcinoma

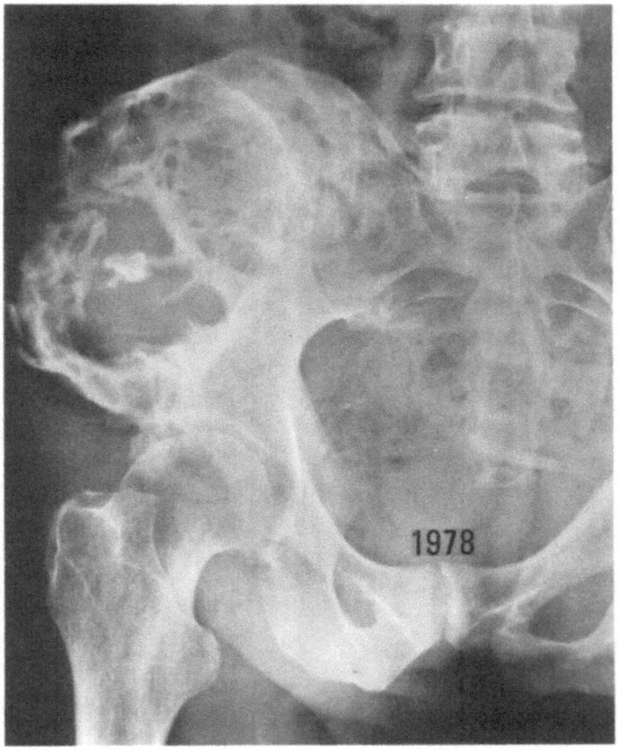

Fig. 11. Radiographic state of healing of same metastasis as in Fig. 10, 3 years later

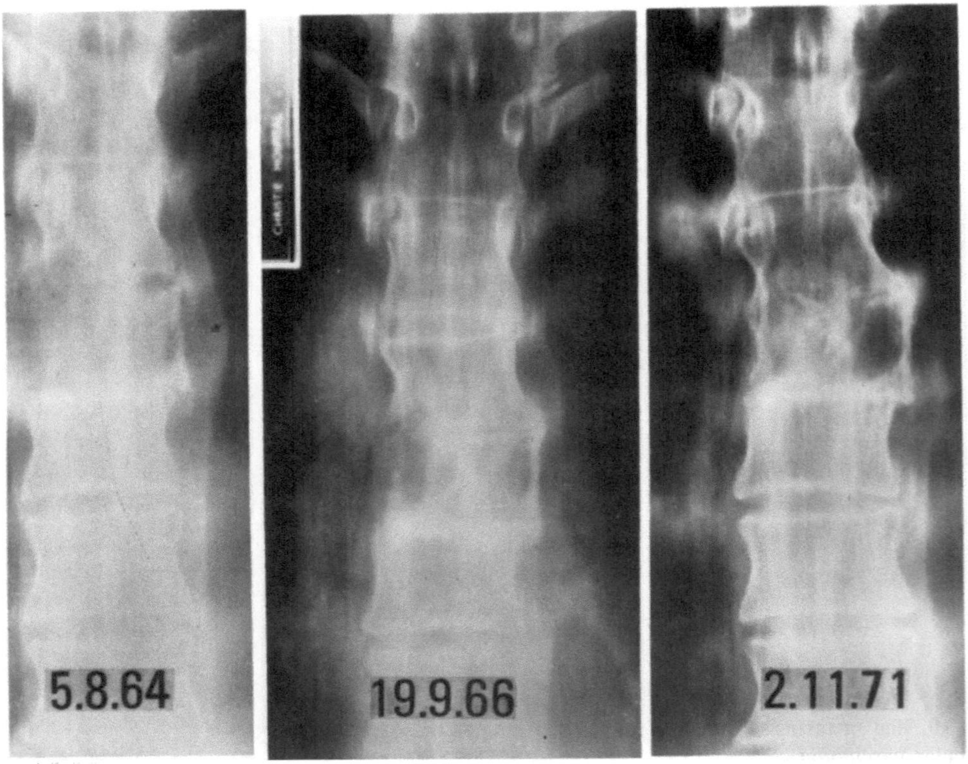

Fig. 12. Spinal metastasis with paraplegia. Full recovery with decompression laminectomy, ^{131}I therapy, and X-ray therapy

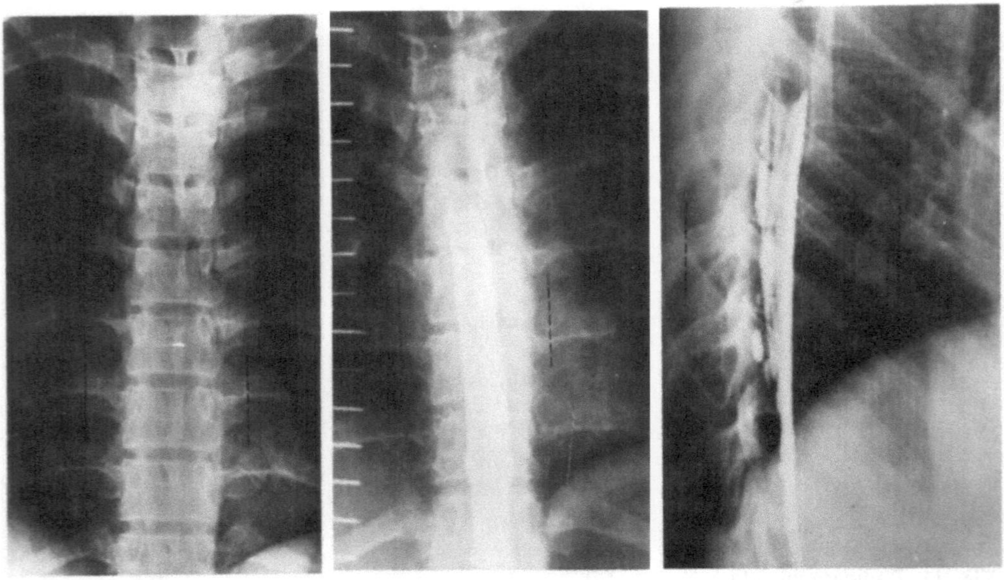

Fig. 13. Paraplegia in the absence of bone involvement. Complete block to intrathecal myodil at T 6

ease in bone (Fig. 12). One recent patient had no X-ray evidence of bone involvement, but myelography showed a total block at T6. Biopsy of a neck mass had revealed anaplastic thyroid carcinoma (Fig. 13).

Liver and Brain

Secondary disease in the liver and the brain may be investigated by appropriate noninvasive procedures based on radionuclide scanning or ultrasound, or both. The role of computerized tomography is reviewed later.

Medullary Cancer (MCT)

A specific section is alloted to MCT because it has proved to be one of the more interesting lesions recognized in recent times, and the question as to whether there is a particular role for radiology in its assessment is relevant.

Of a consecutive series of 382 patients with thyroid cancer seen at the Christie Hospital, Manchester, ten (2.6%) had MCT. Other series show an incidence of between 3.5% (Hazard 1959) and 9.4% (Ibanez 1967).

The following particular features that are demonstrable by X-ray techniques have been variously reported, usually in relation to associated disease in other areas.

Keiser et al. (1973) described selective thyroid arteriography in eight cases. Vascular lakes were seen in only one. The others showed multiple avascular areas, which it was felt might possibly be related to the presence of amyloid deposition.

O'Higgins (1973) referred to lymphatic or direct spread of MCT to the mediastinum, sometimes with areas of calcification, which might appear years after the initial diagnosis. This feature should be satisfactorily identified by serial chest radiography. He also commented upon the fact that intestinal barium studies (where diarrhoea was a feature of the disease) revealed no specifically abnormal features – only hypermotility and rapid transit time.

Familial intestinal polyposis with mucocutaneous pigmented naevi (Gardner's syndrome) was reported as occurring in MCT by DeGroot and Stanbury (1975). Examination of the literature shows that the two cases (siblings) reported by Camiel et al. (1968) actually had papillary carcinoma of the thyroid.

Parathyroid hyperplasia does not seem to be associated with bone changes definable on X-ray examination. Nephrocalcinosis has been reported in one patient (Manning et al. 1963).

The radiologist, viewing the chest X-ray in Marfan's syndrome, has the opportunity to draw attention to a thyroid mass indenting the trachea.

The other conditions associated with MCT are identifiable by biochemical analysis – indeed, the diagnosis of MCT itself is supported by the discovery of raised levels of calcitonin in the serum (resting or following provocation) and in the gland.

Raised values of vanillylmandelic acid and catecholamines in the urine suggest the presence of functioning phaeochromocytoma. Taylor (1977) has commented that phaeochromocytomas are usually bilateral, but Graze et al. (1978), reviewing over 100 persons with a family history of MCT, found an adrenal tumour could be on one side only. Therefore, there may be a place for radiological pursuit with nephrotomography, arteriography, venography, with selective sampling, or perirenal pneumography if the biochemistry suggest this diagnosis.

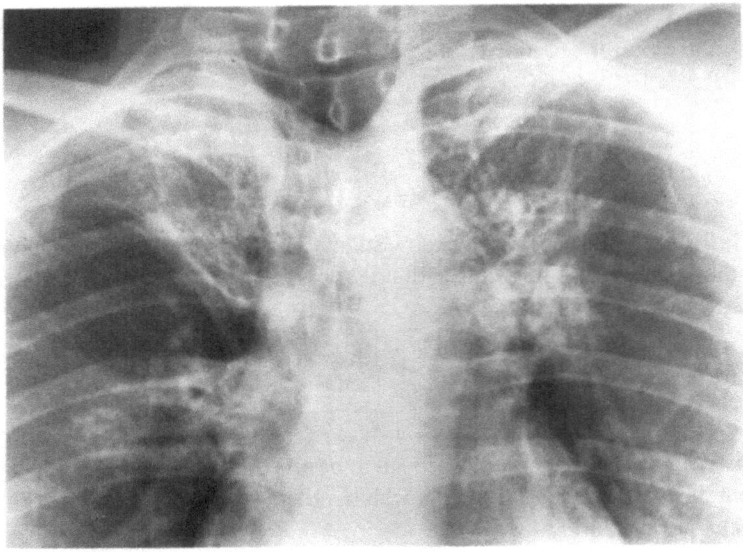

Fig. 14. Pulmonary mediastinal fibrosis after successful X-ray therapy

Inappropriate ACTH secretion will presumably result in bilateral adrenocortical hyperplasia, so that recourse to specific X-ray study is not required. There will be a place, however, for skeletal radiography to determine the presence and degree of osteoporosis, as in the case described by ROSENBERG et al. (1978).

Complications of Radiotherapy

There are two principal complications that concern radiologists:
(1) Radiation fibrosis in the upper mediastinum and adjacent lung (Fig. 14), and
(2) The possiblity of radiation-induced carcinoma of the upper oesophagus where a high total dose was given for thyroid cancer many years earlier (Fig. 15).

The Role of CT Scanning

One current question is whether there is a special place for CT scanning. The following comments are based on experience with a scanner in the investigation of other forms of malignant disease and are derived from its direct application to cancer of the thyroid.

The ability to produce sequential cross-section imaging of the neck should allow a global estimate of the mass lesion and its pressure and invasive effects and demonstration of all calcific opacities with their relation to the tumour.

Serial scanning from the neck into the thorax will reveal, in continuity, the total extension of the primary lesion, with a composite view of the mediastinal and hilar areas and their relationships to one another.

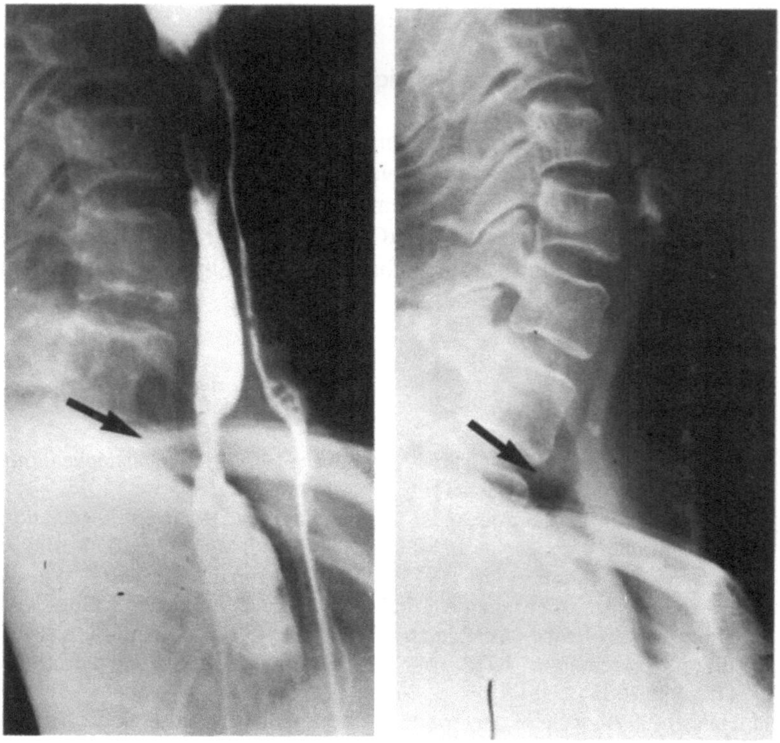

Fig. 15. Upper oesophageal carcinoma occurring 20 years after thyroid irradiation

Within the thorax, *the relation between central and peripheral (pulmonary/pleural) disease* may be shown simultaneously.

The above may be accomplished to some degree by transaxial tomography with radiographic technique, but this does not involve the same facility for interrogation of individual image sections.

Early metastatic lung and pleural disease can be demonstrated better than by conventional radiology.

CT scanning provides an excellent, noninvasive approach to the diagnosis of brain and liver metastases.

It allows convenient demonstration of suprarenal mass lesions, avoiding recourse to invasive procedures.

In chest and abdominal scanning, *it may coincidentally reveal vertebral disease* before clinical suspicion of metastases has been raised.

There is a potential for a *direct link with planning of radiotherapy.*

Conclusions

A multitude of radiological techniques may be applied to the problem of thyroid cancer.

So far as the primary lesion is concerned, the choice of those employed will be influenced by individual clinical attitudes to the investigation of an organ that is readily accessible by more direct methods. In this context it may be apposite to quote ROSENBERG (1972), whose sentiments have been echoed by DEGROOT and STANBURY (1975): "The new and ingenious methods of thyroid study are no substitute for, but may be useful adjuncts to, a thoughtful, clinical appraisal of the case".

References

1 Blum M, Goldman AB, Herskovi A, Hernberg J (1972) Clinical application of thyroid echography. N Engl J Med 287:1164–1169

2 Camiel MR, Mule JE, Alexander LL, Benningham DL (1968) Association of thyroid carcinoma with Gardner's syndrome in siblings. N Engl J Med 278:1056–1068

3 DeGroot LJ, Stanbury JB (1975) The thyroid and its diseases. Wiley & Sons, London

4 Graze K, Spiler IJ, Tashjian AH Jr, Melvin KE, Cervi-Skinner S, Gage RF, Miller HH, Wolfe HJ, DeLellis RA, Leape L, Feldman ZT, Reichlin S (1978) Natural history of familial medullary thyroid carcinoma: effect of a program for early diagnosis. N Engl J Med 299 (18):980–985

5 Hales I (1978) Role of ultrasound in diagnosis of thyroid tumours. In: Hill CR, McCready VR, Cosgrove DO (eds) Ultrasound in tumour diagnosis. Pitman, London

6 Halnan KE, Roberts PH (1967) Paraplegia caused by spinal metastasis from thyroid cancer. Br Med J 3:534–536

7 Hazard JB, Hawk WA, Crile G Jr (1959) Medullary (solid) carcinoma of the thyroid – a clinicopathological entity. J Clin Endocrinol Metab 19:152–161

8 Ibanez ML, Cole VW, Russell WO, Clark R Lee (1967) Solid carcinoma of the thyroid. Cancer 20:706–723

9 Keiser HR, Beaven MA, Doppman J, Wells S, Buja LM (1973) Sipple's syndrome: Medullary thyroid carcinoma, phaechromocytoma and parathyroid disease. Ann Intern Med 78:561–579

10 McDonald J (1970) X-ray diagnosis. In: Smithers DW (ed) Tumours of the thyroid gland. Livingstone, Edinburgh London (Monographs on neoplastic disease), pp 89–201

11 Manning PC, Molnar GD, Black M, Priestley JT, Woolmer LB (1963) Phaechromocytoma, hyperparathyroidism and thyroid carcinoma occurring co-incidentally. New Engl J Med 268:68–72

12 Messaris G, Evangelou GN, Tountas C (1973) Incidence of carcinoma in cold nodules of the thyroid gland. Surgery 74:447–448

13 Miskin M, Rosen IB, Walfish PG (1973) B-mode ultrasonography in assessment of thyroid gland lesions. Ann Intern Med 79:505–510

14 O'Higgins NJ (19737) Medullary thyroid carcinoma. Br J Hosp Med 9:509–519

15 Rosenberg EW, Hahn TJ, Orth DN, Deftos LJ, Tanaka K (1978) ACTH-secreting medullary carcinoma of the thyroid presenting as severe idiopathic osteoporosis and senile purpura: report of a case and review of the literature. J Clin Endocrinol Metab 47:255–262

16 Rosenberg IN (1972) Newer methods for evaluating thyroid nodules. N Engl J Med 287:1197–1198

17 Samuels BI (1972) Thermography: a valuable tool in the detection of thyroid disease. Radiology 102:59–62

18 Sherman RS, Ivker M (1950) The roentgen appearances of thyroid metastases in bone. Am J Roentgenol 63:196–199
19 Takahashi M, Ishibashi T, Kawanami H (1969) Angiographic diagnosis of benign and malignant tumours of the thyroid. Radiology 92:520–526
20 Taylor KJ, Carpenter DA, Barrett JJ (1974) Gray-scale ultrasonography in the diagnosis of thyroid swellings. J Clin Untrasound 2 (4):327–330
21 Taylor S (1958) The thyroid nodule. Lancet 1:751–754
22 Taylor S (1977) Bradshaw Lecture 1976. Thyroid medullary carcinoma. Ann R Coll Surg Engl 59:374–382
23 Thijs LG (1971) Diagnostic ultrasound in clinical thyroid investigation. J Clin Endocrinol Metab 32:709–716
24 Vander JB, Gaston EA, Dawber TR (1968) The significance of nontoxic thyroid nodules. Ann Intern Med 69:537–540
25 Williams ED (1970) Medullary carcinoma. In: Smithers DW (ed) Tumours of the thyroid gland. Livingstone, Edinburgh London (Monographs on neoplastic disease), pp 130–140

Surgical Management

S. Taylor and K. Al-Wattar

Department of Surgery, Royal Postgraduate Medical School, Hammersmith Hospital, GB-London W12 OHS

Introduction

From 1951 to 1975, 355 patients with thyroid malignancy were treated at Hammersmith Hospital. The classification developed by the American Thyroid Association has been used as far as possible (Woolner et al. 1968), and previous to this the classification of Warren and Meissner (1953), the main difference in the former being the recognition of medullary carcinoma as a specific entity and the subdivision of follicular lesions into encapsulated and invasive. The distribution of these tumours by histological type is given in Table 1. The follow-up has extended to the present time, except for those patients with carcinoma who were treated by radiotherapy alone and were referred from other hospitals. The hormone therapy given consisted of thyroxine 0.2 mg daily, and occasionally 0.3 mg daily, and in a few patients triiodothyronine (80–100 μg daily).

The pattern of age and sex of patients presenting with thyroid malignancy differed considerably from the general run of those attending the thyroid clinic. There were 87 males and 268 females, a female : male ratio of almost 3 : 1, whereas in other thyroid diseases there was a of female-to-male ratio of approximately 7 : 1.

Figure 1 shows the sex and age distribution of differentiated carcinoma of the thyroid gland, while Fig. 2 shows the sex and age distribution of anaplastic carcinoma of the thyroid gland.

The various pathological types of carcinoma of the thyroid appeared to occur in characteristic age groups. On the whole, papillary carcinoma was encountered in younger patients (Fig. 3), and all the thyroid carcinomas seen in childhood except one were of this histological type. However, there was a good follicular component in these tumours but the presence of papillary areas placed them in this pathological group in accordance with the American Thyroid Association classification.

Table 1. Incidences and sex ratios of different pathological types encountered in 355 malignant thyroid tumours

Type of tumour	No. of cases	%	Females	Males	Sex ratio
Papillary	133	37.7	94	39	3 : 1
Follicular	75	21.1	57	18	3.2 : 1
Medullary	28	8.1	15	13	1.2 : 1
Anaplastic	97	27.3	82	15	4.5 : 1
Miscellaneous	23	6.1	–	–	–

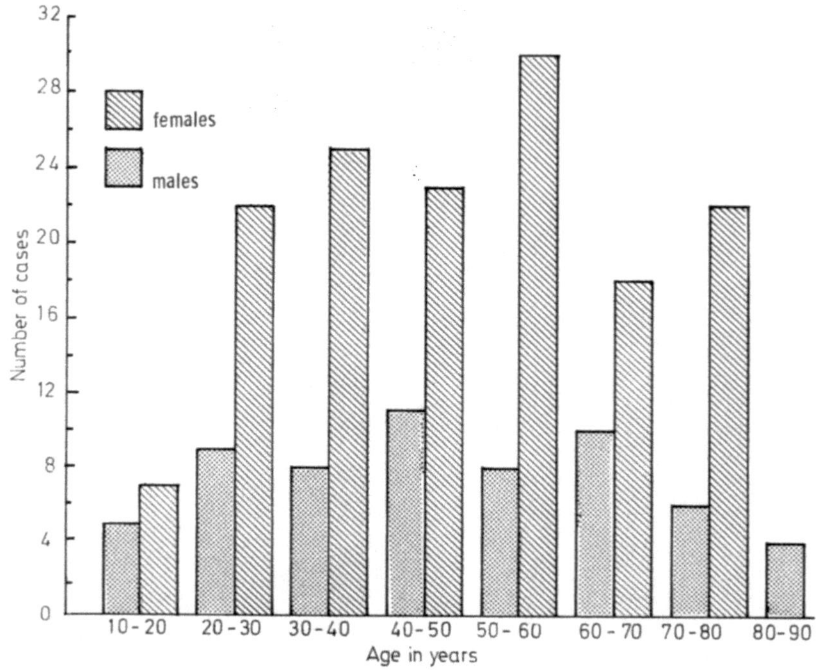

Fig. 1. Age and sex distribution of 355 cases of thyroid carcinoma

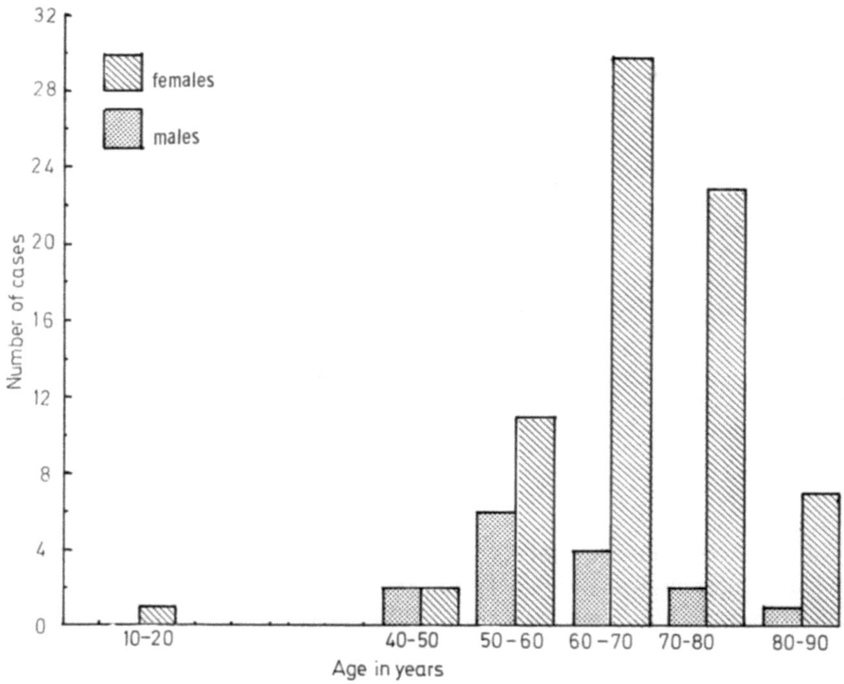

Fig. 2. Age distribution among 89 patients with anaplastic carcinoma

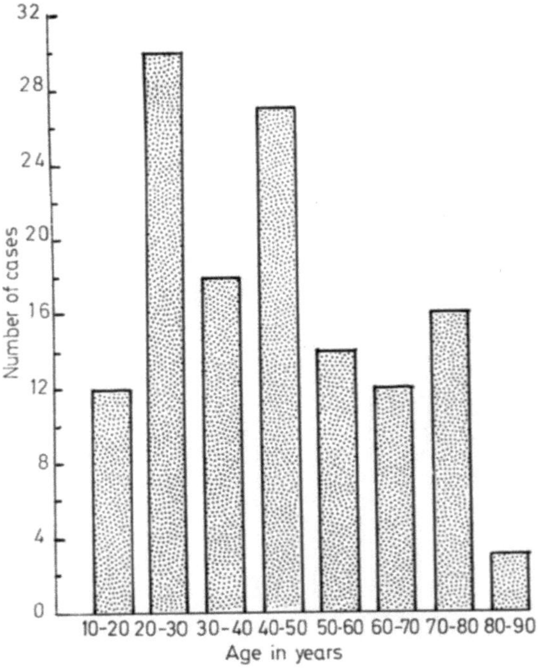

Fig. 3. Age distribution among 133 patients (39 male and 94 female) with papillary carcinoma

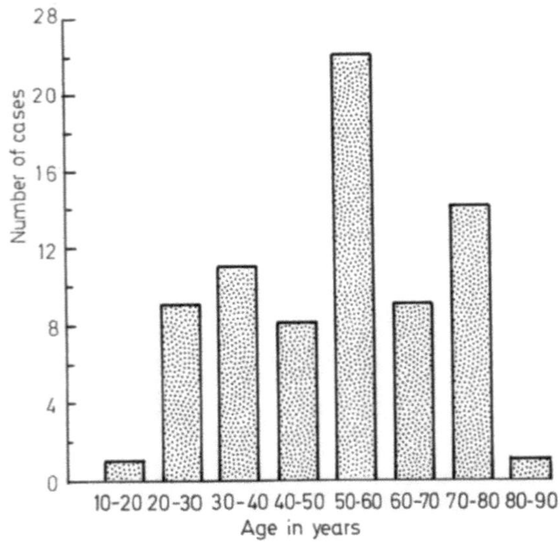

Fig. 4. Age distribution among 75 patients (18 male and 57 female) with follicular carcinoma

Figure 4 shows that the patients with follicular carcinoma, i.e., carcinoma with a purely follicular morphology, were somewhat older.

It will be seen in Fig. 5 that anaplastic carcinoma tended to occur most often after the age of 50. Indeed, there was a preponderance of women over 65. There was no distinctive pattern of age at presentation in medullary carcinoma (Fig. 6). The overall age distribution among 327 patients with thyroid cancer is shown in Fig. 7.

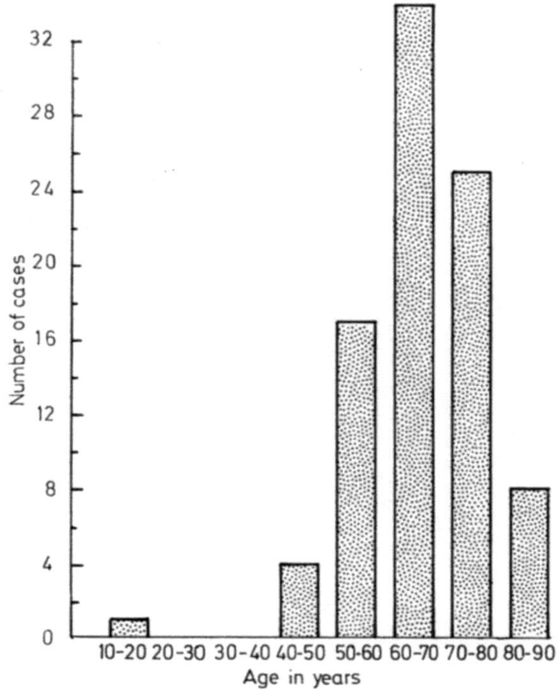

Fig. 5. Age distribution among 89 patients with anaplastic carcinoma

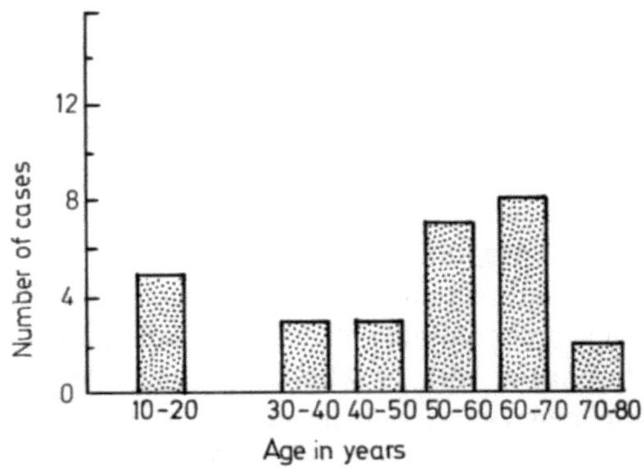

Fig. 6. Age distribution among 28 patients (13 male and 15 female) with MCT

Clinical Presentation

Thyroid carcinoma presented in one of the following ways:

1) A nodule or diffuse enlargement of the gland without other signs or symptoms (approximately 50%),
2) a nodule with enlarged cervical lymph nodes,
3) a nodule with skeletal metastases,
4) a nodule with pulmonary metastases,
5) a nodule with hoarseness of the voice, dyspnoea, dysphagia, and occasionally pain, particularly in the undifferentiated group,
6) a gland that felt normal on palpation, but with evidence of lymph node involvement, recurrent nerve damage, or distant metastases.

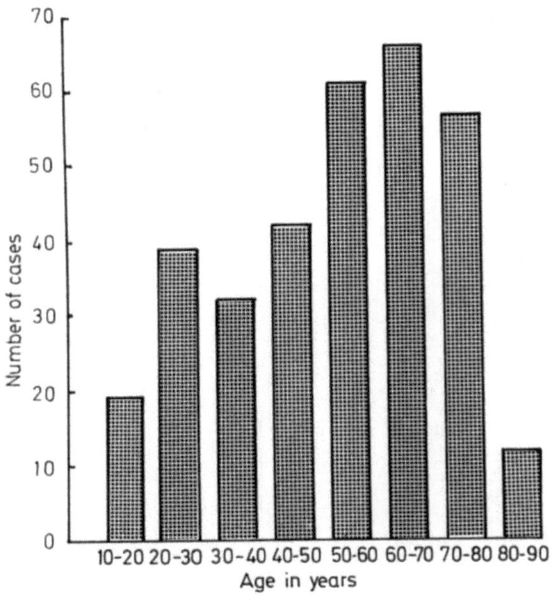

Fig. 7. Overall age distribution of patients with thyroid carcinoma (327 cases)

Four patients first presented with hoarseness of the voice as the only abnormality. Two hundred and sixteen of the 355 patients (about 60%) showed evidence of local or distant spread when they first presented. The metastatic spread of the disease in each group is shown in Table 2, some patients presenting with tumour that had spread by more than one route.

The pattern of spread was characteristic of the tumour type. Papillary carcinoma metastasized in the first place to the local lymph nodes and showed the slowest progression of all the tumour types. Follicular carcinoma disseminated typically by the bloodstream and its behaviour was much less predictable.

Anaplastic carcinoma nearly always spread by direct extension locally into the tissues of the neck, and presented mainly as an enlarging mass with pain, change of voice, dyspnoea, and dysphagia, with or without lymph node involvement or distant spread.

Medullary carcinoma usually spread to the local lymph nodes in the first instance, but it also metastasized later to the skeleton, lungs, and soft tissues (TAYLOR 1977; O'HIGGINS 1973).

Table 2. Metastatic spread of different types of thyroid carcinoma

Spread	Papillary	Follicular	Medullary	Anaplastic
Direct	22	14	3	75
Lymphatic	56	17	14	35
Pulmonary	7	10	2	8
Skeletal	5	12	2	4
	73 of 133	39 of 75	15 of 28	89 of 97

Management

In the treatment of these patients it was useful to simplify the classification of thyroid carcinoma into two main groups, the differentiated, which includes papillary, follicular, and medullary carcinomas, and the undifferentiated group, which includes both the anaplastic carcinomas, and the malignant lymphomas (DUNHILL 1931).

The undifferentiated group had a poor prognosis, and whenever the diagnosis of undifferentiated carcinoma was made clinically in these patients a needle or drill biopsy was carried out. If this confirmed the diagnosis the patient proceeded directly to radiotherapy, major surgery being avoided.

The extremely slow growth of the papillary and some follicular tumours permitted radical excision even when a swelling had been noted in the thyroid gland for many years. It was also apparent on review of these patients' records that follicular carcinoma was first seen in an older age group than the papillary tumours.

The management of thyroid carcinoma can be considered under the following headings:

1) The solitary nodule (the diagnosis of carcinoma being suspected but not confirmed until histological examination later),

2) operation when carcinoma is known to be present (a biopsy or involved lymph node having provided a firm diagnosis).

The Solitary Nodule

Whenever a solitary nodule was seen or palpated, particularly when it was cold on scan, it was excised. None in this series was less than 2 cm in diameter. The younger the patient, the likelier was the diagnosis to be carcinoma. The treatment in such patients was total excision of the lobe containing the nodule and preservation of the parathyroid glands and recurrent nerve. Even when a parathyroid gland was removed it caused no more than temporary hypocalcaemia, and sometimes not even that, presumably because the parathyroids on the other side of the neck were not disturbed.

Once the histological diagnosis was established, and 13% of all our clinically solitary nodules were malignant (TAYLOR and PSARRAS 1967), the patient was given thyroxine orally with the aim of suppressing the TSH, which was regarded as one of the stimuli for growth of any metastases that might be present (TAYLOR 1963). It was not the practice in this series to follow

Table 3. Pathology of 207 clinically solitary nodules

Classification	Nodularity		Total
	Single	Multiple	
Benign	94	87	181
Malignant	14	12	26 = 12.6%
	108	99	207

these lobectomies by radiotherapy, but the patients were examined at regular intervals (at first every 6 months and later annually), so that any increase in size of the remaining thyroid tissue and the appearance of any involved lymph nodes could be detected and further surgery carried out. These patients received thyroxine for the rest of their lives. Table 3 gives the pathology of 207 solitary nodules.

Proven Carcinoma

When carcinoma was known to be present because an involved lymph node had already been removed, total thyroidectomy was the next step in treatment, with the local removal of any apparently involved lymph nodes. If the strap muscles were involved they were excised in continuity with the tumour, preserving the recurrent nerves and retaining the parathyroids, except when they were involved by the carcinoma. If, however, no involved nodes were seen, the usual practice was to prescribe thyroxine and examine the patient at intervals to see whether further disease appeared.

Particular attention was directed to the removal of the involved lymph nodes (TAYLOR 1964). Unlike most lymph node metastases encountered in the neck, the nodes involved by papillary carcinoma were very mobile and could be removed individually. Formal block dissection was never performed, but when the tumour or nodes adhered to the muscle this was excised in continuity. Trachea was also locally excised if involved. The jugular vein was only removed when malignant nodes appeared to invade its wall.

In patients in whom follicular carcinoma had metastasized to the bones or lungs, radioiodine was given and the body scanned. The best results were obtained in patients whose secondaries took up some of the isotope even before total thyroidectomy. Postoperatively, during the early days of treating thyroid cancer, the metastases were further stimulated to metabolize iodine by allowing the patient to develop myxoedema. More recently this method of stimulation has been superseded by IM injection of 10 U TSH before a tracer dose of ^{131}I. If the secondaries took up the radioiodine, a large therapeutic dose of isotope was given (normally 200 mCi).

For patients with undifferentiated carcinoma confirmed by drill or needle biopsy, the usual procedure was local radiotherapy and hormonal replacement. Some patients presented in similar fashion but were found to have malignant lymphoma. It is of interest to note that the best response to radiotherapy was seen in these patients with malignant lymphoma, who had a relatively longer survival than those with anaplastic carcinoma (TAYLOR 1974).

Results of Treatment

For various reasons, 13 patients with differentiated carcinoma were not seen after their discharge from the hospital, and eventually 33 patients could not be traced. All these were recorded in Fig. 7 as dead, and the prognosis therefore appears much worse than it should. A number of patients died of intercurrent disease.

In papillary carcinoma the survival was better than in all the other groups.

In patients with follicular carcinoma, two distinct prognostic groups emerged, depending on the clinical presentation and pathological findings of the tumour. In one group, examination of the tumour showed no capsular or vascular invasion and in the second group there was either capsular or vascular invasion or both. Clinically, tumours of the second group showed more rapid growth of the swelling in the neck and tended to metastasize to the lungs and skeleton.

Medullary carcinoma was a distinct variant (HAZARD et al. 1959); which occurred sporadically but can be found affecting certain families as one part of the syndrome of multiple endocrine adenomatosis (MEA) type 2, when it may be accompanied by bilateral phaeochromocytomas and parathyroid hyperplasia or adenoma (HARRISON and THOMSON 1975). In some patients it was associated with multiple neuromas of the eyelids and tongue and the individuals showed a Marfan-like habitus, a syndrome now called MEA 2b; all three of these cases in our series were sporadic and not familial (TAYLOR 1977). Some patients with medullary carcinoma had diarrhoea, the cause of which is obscure, but removal of a large part of the tumour mass relieved it. The use of nutmeg did not help these patients.

The histology of these tumours was distinguished by the presence of amyloid in the stroma and sometimes the cells appeared very malignant, closely resembling those found in fibrosarcomas. Despite this histological appearance, these tumours proved to be among the slowest-growing of the thyroid cancers observed in this series, some only spreading to the mediastinum after a period of more than 20 years. Previously this tumour had been diagnosed in our patients as anaplastic because of its histological appearance. Medullary carcinoma remains unique among thyroid tumours in affecting both sexes equally.

This type of carcinoma was characterized by high levels of calcitonin in the serum of the affected patients (CUNLIFFE et al. 1968; JACKSON et al. 1973). Radioimmunoassay of calcitonin was used both as a marker in diagnosis and also to follow the progress of the patient after surgery. None of our medullary tumours that were irradiated appeared to be particularly radiosensitive. These carcinomas do not concentrate radioiodine, being derived from the C cells of the neural ectoderm (WILLIAMS 1972) and so radioiodine played no part in their treatment.

Anaplastic carcinoma is one of the most aggressive of all malignant tumours. It killed many patients in a few months and few survived for 1 year. Diagnosis was confirmed in most of them by drill biopsy, and neither subtotal nor total thyroidectomy was attempted. Radiotherapy provided the best palliation, treatment being given not only to the neck but also to the upper mediastinum through a variety of fields. Regression often occurred initially with this treatment. It was the malignant lymphomas that responded best to radiotherapy, however, with an average survival of 3 years.

Miscellaneous Tumours of the Thyroid

Few cases of thyroid sarcoma were seen, either of the reticulum-cell variety or of the fibrosarcoma type. The reticulum-cell variety responded well to radiotherapy, but recurred and progressed rapidly. Twe cases of fibrosarcoma developed in toxic goitres treated with radioiodine, but it was considered improbable that this was a factor in their causation.

Four cases of squamous-cell carcinoma were seen. It was assumed that these were formed by squamous metaplasia in papillary thyroid tumours.

One patient was found to have a malignant teratoma of the thyroid. The tumour was very aggressive and despite excision of nodes, radiotherapy, and chemotherapy the patient died within a few months.

Examples of tumours metastasizing to the thyroid were seen sporadically. The usual primary sites were the ovary, kidney, pharynx, and melanoma.

Conclusions

Patients with thyroid tumour referred to our clinic have been reviewed at intervals (ALHADEFF et al. 1956; BURN and TAYLOR 1962; TAYLOR and DAVIS 1970) and now in 1976, thus making it possible to note changes in both the pattern of disease and its treatment over a period of some 30 years.

The ratio of differentiated to undifferentiated thyroid cancer has risen from 1 : 1 to 2.5 : 1 in this time. This is in part due to the recognition of medullary carcinoma as an entity in 1959, since this was often labelled undifferentiated before that date and is now clearly seen to be relatively slow-growing and differentiated. What other factors are at work is pure surmise.

This review confirms the prognostic value of the size of the primary tumour, histology, and age at presentation, and shows that the presence of papillary node metastases is compatible with long survival.

Nodules that are solitary on clinical examination, and especially those that are cold on scanning, have been seen to harbour differentiated carcinoma in 10%–20% of patients in many countries. The incidence of cancer in solitary nodules in our clinic was 13%. Many grow slowly and may not affect the normal lifespan of the patient. On the other hand, it may be that their removal has helped to lower the overall number of anaplastic carcinomas, since the workers at the MD Anderson Hospital at Houston have convincingly demonstrated that most, if not all, anaplastic thyroid tumours arise from differentiated ones (RUSSELL et al. 1968).

Ionizing radiation in small doses has been shown to be carcinogenic in the thyroid gland during infancy and childhood (DUFFY and FITZGERALD 1950; HEMPELMANN 1968). The latent period before development of a clinically recognized tumour may be 20 years, and this type of tumour has reached epidemic proportions in recent years (DEGROOT et al. 1977).

The value of thyroxine therapy in suppressing the pituitary stimulus to tumour growth has become universally recognized, and all our patients are maintained on thyroxine.

Thyroxine also finds a special place in the control of thyroid carcinoma in children in whom the tumours seem to be hormone-dependent. Three of our patients are now adults who lead normal lives despite evidence of multiple pulmonary metastases that have shrunk but not disappeared over the years. Suppression of TSH seems to be the critical factor, and the dose of thyroxine has been adjusted until TSH is barely detectable by radioimmunoassay.

The use of radiotherapy has been largely restricted in recent years to the treatment of anaplastic thyroid carcinoma and malignant lymphoma, and we do not yet know whether it may be of value in medullary carcinoma. The only tumours responding to radioiodine therapy were follicular in pattern and there were remarkably few patients in our series who showed significant clinical improvement in response to radioiodine.

Thyroid cancer accounts for only 10% of all neoplasms. Differentiated thyroid tumours are rare and slow-growing, so that the pattern of treatment evolves very gradually. Over the last 25 years there has certainly been a swing to a more conservative surgical approach in our clinic. Further study requires continuing long-term multicentre collaboration.

Acknowledgements. We are particularly grateful for the assistance, past and present, of many colleagues. For assistance in pathology, we mention especially I. DONIACH, D. WILLIAMS, and P. LEWIS. A. W. G. GOOLDEN provided all the radiotherapy and isotope therapy and referred many of the patients for surgical treatment.

References

1 Alhadeff R, Scott F, Taylor S (1956) A clinico-pathological study of thyroid carcinoma. Br J Surg 43:617–626
2 Burn JI, Taylor S (1962) The natural history of thyroid carcinoma. A study of 152 treated patients. Br Med J 2:1218–1220
3 Cunliffe WJ, Black MM, Hall R, Johnston IDA, Hudgson P, Shuster S, Gudmundsson TV, Joplin GF, Williams ED, Woodhouse NJY, Galante L, MacIntyre I (1968) A calcitonin-secreting thyroid carcinoma. Lancet 2:63–66
4 DeGroot LJ, Frohmen LA, Kaplan EL, Refetoss S (1977) Radiation-associated thyroid carcinoma. Grune & Stratton, New York
5 Duffy BJ Jr, Fitzgerald BJ (1950) Cancer of the thyroid in children: A report of 28 cases. J Clin Endocrinol Metab 10:1296
6 Dunhill TP (1931) Carcinoma of the thyroid gland. Br J Surg 19:83–113
7 Harrison TS, Thomson NW (1975) Multiple endocrine adenomatosis, I and II. Year Book, Chicago, (Current problems in surgery)
8 Hazard JB, Hawk WA, Crile G Jr (1959) Medullary (solid) carcinoma of the thyroid, a clinicopathological entity. J Clin Endocrinol Metab 19:152–161
9 Hempelmann LH (1968) Radiation induced neoplasms in man. In: S Young, Inman DR (eds) Thyroid neoplasia. Academic Press, London, pp 267–276
10 Jackson CE, Tashjian AH, Black AM (1973) Detection of medullary carcinoma by calcitonin assay in families. Ann Intern Med 78:845–852
11 O'Higgins NJ (1973) Medullary carcinoma of the thyroid. Br J Hosp Med 9:509–519
12 Russel WO, Ibanez ML, Stratton-Hill C Jr, Clark RL, White EC (1968) Papillary and follicular thyroid carcinoma: prognostic significance of the type variation in 97 of 116 primary tumours studied by whole organ sections. In: S Joung, Inman DR (eds) Thyroid neoplasia. Academic Press, London, pp 109–132
13 Taylor S (1963) Limitations of thyrotropin suppression in the treatment of nodular goiter and thyroid carcinoma. In: Werner SC (ed) Thyrotropin. Thomas, Springfield Illinois, pp 353–358
14 Taylor S (1964) Indications and technique for lymph node surgery in tumours of the thyroid gland. In: Appaix A (ed) International colloquium for tumours of the thyroid gland, Marseille. Karger, Basel New York, p 426
15 Taylor S (1974) Thyroid cancer, surgical methods and treatment – Their indications and value. Proc R Soc Med 67:1105–1106
16 Taylor S (1977) Thyroid medullary carcinoma. Ann R Coll Surg Engl 59:374–381
17 Taylor S, Davis PW (1970) A review of the treatment of 222 patients with malignant tumours of the thyroid gland. In: Smithers DW (ed) Tumours of the thyroid gland. Livingstone, Edinburgh, pp 243–258
18 Warren S, Meissner WA (1953) Tumours of the thyroid gland. Armed Forces Institute of Pathology, Washington DC Fasc. 14
19 Woolner LB, Beahrs OH, Black BM, McConahey WM, Keating FR Jr (1968) General considerations and value of data on 1181 cases – Long term survival rates. In: S Young, Inman DR (eds) Thyroid neoplasia. Academic Press, London, pp 51–79

Radiotherapy

A. W. G. Goolden

Department of Radiotherapy and Oncology, Royal Postgraduate Medical School
and Hammersmith Hospital, GB-London W12 OHS

Introduction

Although the stage of the disease has clearly to be taken into account, the management of patients with malignant disease of the thyroid gland depends largely on the pathological diagnosis. It is appropriate therefore, before discussing treatment, to look at the histological classification of thyroid tumours (Table 1).

Classification of Thyroid Tumours

The differentiated thyroid tumours arise from the follicular cells. They have been divided into papillary and follicular subtypes. The papillary tumours have been further subdivided into occult, intrathyroidal, and extrathyroidal, the last term denoting that the thyroid capsule has been breached. Follicular tumours have been subdivided into microangioinvasive, where spread is restricted to the capsular venous sinuses, and angioinvasive, where the tumour has extended into the extracapsular veins. The subdivision of follicular tumours into microangioinvasive and angioinvasive is in accordance with the classification adopted by Woolner et al. (1961) and Hazard (1964), but many pathologists might find it difficult to make this dis-

Table 1. Classification of thyroid tumours

Follicular cell origin		
Differentiated carcinoma		
	Papillary	Occult
		Intrathyroidal
		Extrathyroidal
	Follicular	Microangioinvasive
		Angioinvasive
Undifferentiated carcinoma		
	Anaplastic carcinoma	
Parafollicular cell origin		
	Medullary carcinoma	
Lymphoreticular cell origin		
	Malignant lymphoma	

tinction and prefer simply to comment on the degree of differentiation and invasiveness of the tumour.

The undifferentiated or anaplastic carcinomas also arise from the follicular cells, and there is now good evidence to support the concept that most of these tumours arise in pre-existing well-differentiated thyroid carcinomas (NISHIYAMA et al. 1972; ALDINGER et al. 1978). There has been some difficulty in the past in the classification of lymphomas of the thyroid. Previously many small-cell tumours were regarded as anaplastic carcinomas, but there has been an increasing tendency during the past 20 years to diagnose these tumours as malignant lymphomas. Medullary carcinoma of the thyroid (MCT), first described as a distinct clinico-pathological entity by HAZARD et al. (1959), is now known to arise from the parafollicular or C cells.

Management of Differentiated Tumours

The treatment of differentiated tumours of the thyroid is primarily by surgery, but radiotherapy with either external irradiation or radioiodine is frequently employed as ancillary treatment. The role of radiotherapy and the results of treatment in patients with well-differentiated thyroid tumours are not well documented, and practice seems to vary from one centre to another. It is commonly believed that differentiated thyroid tumours are resistant to external irradiation. This may be true for papillary carcinoma, although facts and figures are hard to come by, but it is not true for follicular tumours, which may resolve completely after radiotherapy (Fig. 1). Before deciding whether to give radiotherapy, it is clearly important to take into consideration the pathological type and the extent of the disease, and whether or not the tumour is thought to have been completely removed by surgery.

Most differentiated carcinomas contain both papillary and follicular components. All degrees of transition, from purely papillary to purely follicular, are seen. The term "mixed papillary

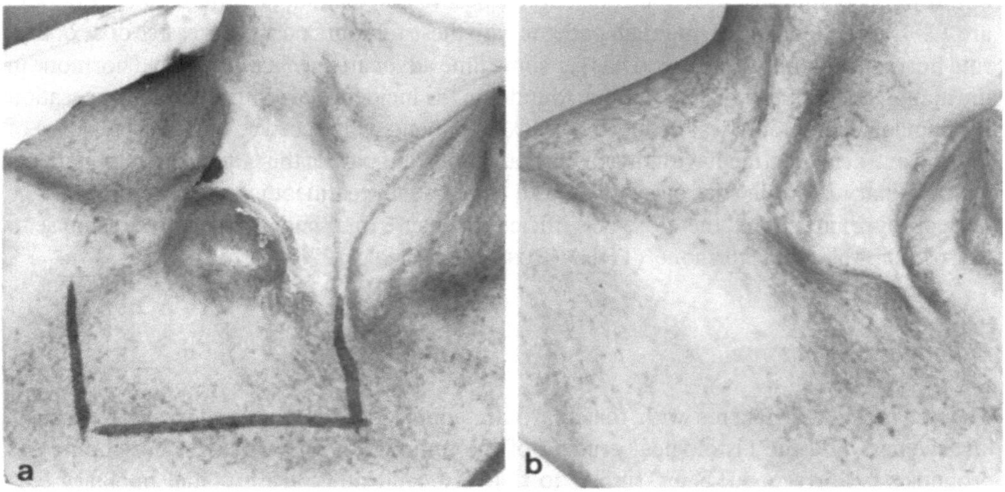

Fig. 1a, b. Recurrence in a patient with follicular thyroid carcinoma before treatment (**a**) and 6 months after a course of external irradiation (**b**)

and follicular" has often been used and could well be applied to the majority of differentiated tumours. If, however, a papillary pattern is seen the tumour will tend to behave as a papillary carcinoma and should be classified as such. A correct diagnosis is important because papillary carcinoma is a curable disease. Although the prognosis is very good for the majority of patients, the outlook is less favourable for those over the age of 40.

Papillary Carcinoma

Patients with occult or intrathyroidal tumours are unlikely to have a recurrence after lobectomy, despite the high incidence of widespread microscopic foci reported in one series (RUSSELL et al. 1963). Long-term survival data from the Mayo Clinic have shown that these patients have a normal expectation of life (WOOLNER et al. 1969). Extrathyroidal papillary tumours, on the other hand, are more malignant and require a total thyroidectomy, with removal of lymph nodes if these are involved. Total removal of all thyroid tissue is difficult to achieve, however, and attempts may result in hypoparathyroidism or damage to the recurrent laryngeal nerve. In this situation, destruction of all normal thyroid tissue can be effected by giving radioiodine postoperatively. If removal of the tumour itself is thought to have been incomplete external irradiation should also be considered.

It is of interest, and relevant to the management of patients with papillary carcinoma, to know whether these tumours concentrate iodine and to what extent they are TSH-dependent. If thyroid tissue is examined by autoradiography, radioactivity is seen to be confined to the colloid contained within the follicle. It is not seen in the cells lining the follicle. It is doubtful whether differentiated tumours concentrate iodine to any significant extent unless they contain colloid, and hence some follicular component. The observation that papillary tumours concentrate iodine is probably based on the fact that many of these tumours have a mixed papillary and follicular structure. Purely papillary tumours are probably incapable of thyroid hormone biosynthesis.

The question of hormone dependence is a little more difficult to answer. TSH stimulation of growth and function in a tumour may also depend on the presence of a follicular component, but from the point of view of management it is best to assume that all differentiated tumours are TSH-dependent and to maintain patients with these tumours on a suppressive dose of thyroid hormone. CRILE (1968), who has for some time advocated the use of thyroid hormone in the management of thyroid carcinoma, found that the incidence of recurrence after operation for papillary carcinoma was reduced by 50% in patients who received suppressive doses of thyroid extract. Treatment with thyroxine is an important part of the management of patients with papillary and follicular carcinoma. The aim of such treatment is to suppress TSH. The dose of thyroxine should therefore be sufficient to ensure that there is a negative response to thyrotropin-releasing hormone (TRH) (BUSNARDO et al. 1976).

Follicular Carcinoma

The prognosis for patients with follicular carcinoma depends on the degree of vascular invasiveness and the histological grading of the tumour. In microinvasive carcinoma the prognosis is fairly good, being similar to that of occult and intrathyroidal papillary carcinoma. Some surgeons perform a lobectomy for these tumours, with or without subtotal resection on the opposite side. Others do a total thyroidectomy. There is a good case for ablating any thyroid remnant with radioiodine, provided that residual thyroid tissue can be demonstrated by scanning, because these tumours are potentially functioning and may already have metastasized. VARMA et al. (1970) reported a significant improvement in survival in patients over the age of 40 with differentiated tumours who were given ^{131}I after surgery. They advised ^{131}I ablation of residual thyroid tissue for all patients with differentiated tumours, papillary as well as follicular. An argument in favour of such a policy is that treatment given prophylactically stands a better chance of success than treatment given at a later stage when there is obvious recurrence. Radiation, in common with other therapeutic methods, is more likely to be effective when microscopic foci rather than large tumour masses are treated.

The treatment of angioinvasive carcinoma needs to be more radical, and there is general agreement that a total thyroidectomy is the operation of choice for patients with such tumours. Uptake of ^{131}I can usually be demonstrated by thyroid scanning, even in patients who have had a so-called total thyroidectomy. Here again, ^{131}I ablation of the thyroid remnant is probably advisable, and will facilitate both the detection and treatment of any functioning metastases that may subsequently develop. HENK et al. (1972) has recommended that a whole-body scan be performed after thyroid ablation, since a substantial number of patients with differentiated tumours were shown by this investigation to have occult metastases. These were usually located in the lungs, and uptake ceased after treatment with ^{131}I.

If surgical removal is known to have been incomplete further treatment is required. In most cases this will include external irradiation; but the possibility that follicular tumours may concentrate iodine must be borne in mind, and treatment with ^{131}I should therefore be considered in addition to external irradiation. The difficulty here is that some normal thyroid tissue will almost certainly have been left behind and if the neck is scanned, it may not be possible to distinguish uptake of ^{131}I in tumour from that in normal thyroid tissue. This problem can usually be resolved by giving an ablative dose of ^{131}I to destroy all normal thyroid tissue, and carrying out a further investigation 3 months later. If any focal concentration of istope is seen it can be assumed that this represents functioning tumour rather than normal thyroid tissue, in which case further treatment with ^{131}I is indicated. In the meantime, external irradiation can be undertaken and will not interfere with any ^{131}I therapy that may be required subsequently, because the maximum dose that can be given by convential radiotherapy is unlikely to have any significant effect on thyroid function.

External irradiation is also indicated in patients with differentiated tumours that are inoperable in the first place and in patients who develop a recurrence, unless complete surgical excision is likely to be achieved by a further operation. SMEDAL et al. (1967) found that both papillary and follicular tumours responded well to irradiation: the 5-year survival rate for patients with nonresectable disease treated by external irradiation was 82%. Here also ^{131}I should be used in addition to external irradiation to ablate normal thyroid tissue and to treat the primary tumour if it concentrates iodine.

Treatment Techniques

External Beam Irradiation

External irradiation may be directed to the thyroid in the form of X-rays by means of megavoltage equipment or as gamma rays derived from a ^{60}Cobalt source. The anatomical situation of the thyroid gland and its regional lymph nodes in relation to the spinal cord makes radiotherapy in this area technically difficult, because the relatively high dose required for dif-

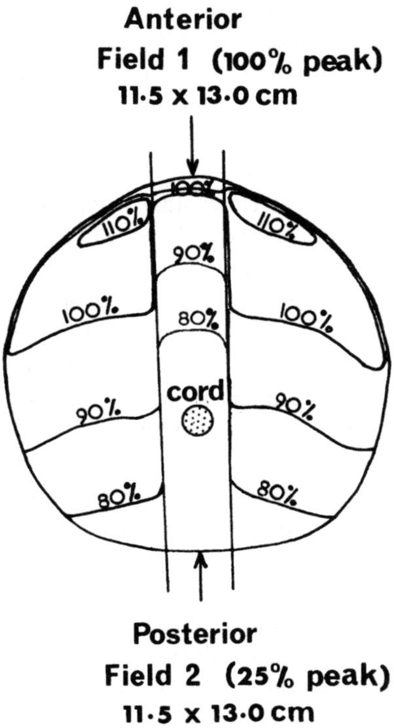

Fig. 2. Dose distribution from telecobalt unit when anterior and posterior opposed fields are used, with shielding to reduce the dose to the spinal cord from the posterior field

ferentiated thyroid tumours, if delivered to the spinal cord, could result in radiation myelitis.

For disease that is confined to the region of the thyroid gland and the immediately adjacent lymph nodes on one or both sides of the neck, treatment can be given through two opposed lateral fields compensated with wedge filters to allow for the contour of the neck and arranged so that their posterior margins do not extend as far back as the spinal cord. This technique is unsatisfactory if the tumour extends too far posteriorly or if the lowest of the cervical lymph nodes are involved, with the likelihood that the disease has extended into the superior mediastinum. In this situation opposed anterior and posterior fields can be used, with shielding of the spinal cord when treatment is given through the posterior field (Fig. 2). The radiation dose required for differentiated thyroid tumours is about 4500 rads in 4 weeks or its equivalent if a different fractionation scheme is used.

The problems of irradiating the thyroid gland and adjacent nodes can be largely overcome if electrons of about 30 MeV are used, but electrons of this energy can only be obtained from a Betatron or a high-energy linear accelerator. The use of electron beams of different energies makes it possible to give an adequate tumour dose through single anterior fields to both neck and mediastinum, and if wax build-up material is used to compensate in the midline of the cervical field the isodose curve is such that the dose to the spinal cord is reduced to an acceptable level (Harmer 1977).

Radioiodine

About 50% of patients with follicular carcinoma have metastases when first seen, and patients with this variety of thyroid tumour often complain first of symptoms due to metastatic

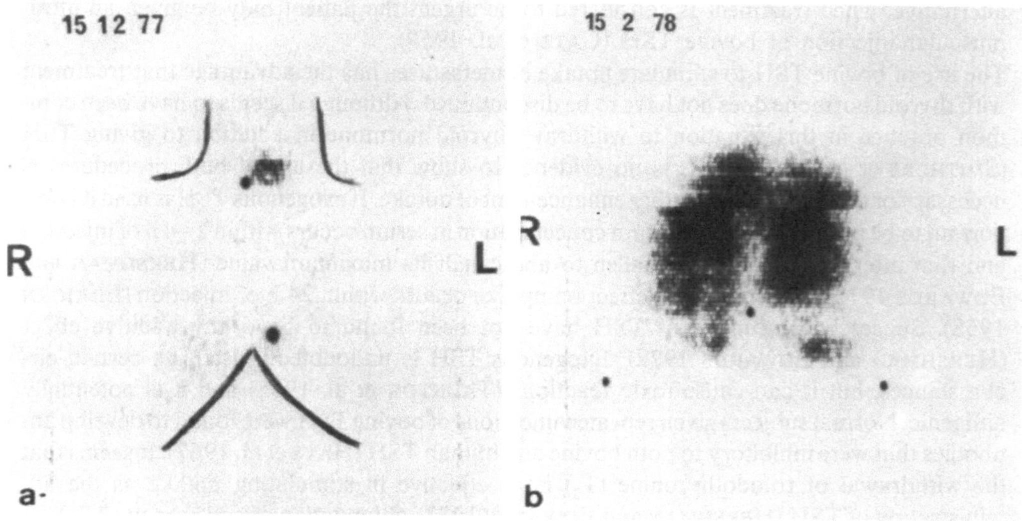

Fig. 3a, b. Photoscans of a patient who had undergone lobectomy for a follicular carcinoma of the thyroid and was subsequently found to have multiple metastases in both lungs before ablation of remaining lobe (**a**) and 2 months later after ^{131}I ablation of normal thyroid tissue (**b**)

disease. The spread is usually to the skeleton or lungs and there may sometimes be a solitary skeletal metastasis.

Any patient who has a metastasis from a follicular carcinoma of the thyroid should be considered as a possible candidate for treatment with radioiodine. It may be possible in some patients to demonstrate function in tumour tissue before the thyroid has been removed. More commonly thyroid ablation must first be carried out, because normal thyroid tissue concentrates iodine more efficiently than even highly differentiated tumour tissue. Surgical ablation of the thyroid is the method of choice, but when the primary tumour is considered to be inoperable or the general condition of the patient is poor the thyroid may be destroyed by radioiodine (Fig. 3).

A radiation dose of at least 50000 rads is needed if ^{131}I is used to ablate the thyroid gland (GOOLDEN and DAVEY 1963). To achieve this dose an initial concentration of 1 mCi ^{131}I per gram of thyroid tissue is required. These considerations apply to destruction of the whole gland or of at least one whole lobe. If it is intended to ablate a small remnant in a patient who has had most of the gland removed, due allowance must be made for the shortened biological half-life of ^{131}I in the residual thyroid tissue. Paradoxically, the smaller the amount of thyroid tissue remaining the more difficult it becomes to destroy it with radioiodine.

After thyroid ablation the patient is allowed to become hypothyroid. The induction of hypothyroidism will be accompanied by an increase in the level of serum TSH, with the result that any tumour tissue that is capable of concentrating iodine will be stimulated to do so. The uptake of radioiodine in tumour tissue may often be further enhanced by giving an antithyroid drug, such as carbimazole. This is likely to be most effective in patients who already have functioning metastases that are producing enough hormone to maintain the patient in an euthyroid or slightly hypothyroid state. The use of an antithyroid drug in these circumstances ensures that the tumour is subjected to maximum TSH stimulation. The induction of hypothyroidism is probably the best means of stimulating thyroid metastases to function, but it does impose some delay in a treatment that tends to be rather protracted in any case. As an alternative, when treatment is considered to be urgent the patient may be given an intramuscular injection of bovine TSH (CATZ et al. 1959).

The use of bovine TSH to stimulate uptake in metastases has the advantage that treatment with thyroid hormone does not have to be discontinued. Although it seems to have been common practice in this situation to withdraw thyroid hormone in addition to giving TSH (SMITHERS et al. 1965), there is no evidence to show that the use of both procedures is necessary or that it results in further enhancement of uptake. If exogenous TSH is used it is important to be aware that its maximum concentration in serum occurs within 2—4 h of injection and that after about 8 h it has fallen to about half its maximum value (HERSHMAN and EDWARDS 1972). The maximum effect on uptake occurs within 24 h of injection (EINHORN 1958). Successive injections of TSH have not been found to have any additive effect (HERSHMAN and EDWARDS 1972). Exogenous TSH is undoubtedly useful in certain circumstances, but it can cause toxic reactions (TAUNTON et al. 1965) and it is potentially antigenic. Normal subjects given repeated injections of bovine TSH were found to develop antibodies that were inhibitory to both bovine and human TSH (HAYS et al. 1967). It seems that the withdrawal of triiodothyronine (T_3) is as effective in stimulating uptake as the administration of TSH (HERSHMAN and EDWARDS 1972). Stimulation of endogenous TSH secretion by the administration of TRH proved ineffective as a means of increasing uptake in patients with thyroid carcinoma (SAMAAN et al. 1972).

It has been recommended that patients with functioning metastases be treated with ^{131}I given at intervals of about 3 months until such time as it is no longer possible to demonstrate uptake in tumour tissue (POCHIN 1967). The usual practice is to give 150—200 mCi. It will be found that progressively smaller amounts of ^{131}I are concentrated in tumour tissue after each therapeutic dose. A whole-body scan is preferable to a profile scan for the demonstration of uptake in metastatic tissue, because a two-dimensional display makes it easier to distinguish uptake in tumour from that in organs such as stomach or liver, which normally concentrate iodine or iodinated compounds. Measurement of the amount of ^{131}I in a metastasis may be achieved either by the profile method (CORBETT et al. 1956) or by means of the two-dimensional display (SCOTT et al. 1970). Calculation of the radiation dose is more difficult, because of uncertainty about the volume of tissue in which the isotope is distributed, but a rough estimate can usually be made. It is unlikely that any therapeutic benefit will be achieved if the concentration of ^{131}I is less than 0.01% of the dose per gram of tumour tissue. At this concentration the radiation dose to the tumour, assuming a biological half-life of 4 days, would amount to no more than 500 rads if the patient were given 150 mCi ^{131}I.

It should be pointed out that a dose of radiation sufficient to destroy the reproductive capacity of a tumour may have little immediate effect on its functional state and that persistent function does not necessarily mean that the tumour is still viable. Tumour regression may be seen in metastases that retain their functional capacity.

Patients undergoing treatment with ^{131}I have to be maintained in the intervals between treatment on thyroid hormone, which has to be stopped before a further dose of ^{131}I is given. In this situation T_3 is preferable to thyroxine, because it has a considerably shorter biological half-life and serum TSH will therefore rise more quickly after discontinuation of T_3 than after T_4 is stopped. At least 2 weeks should be allowed to elapse after the withdrawal of T_3 before tests are carried out; in some patients it may be 3 weeks or more before the serum TSH reaches maximum values (HERSHMAN and EDWARDS 1972). The maintenance dose of T_3 in the intervals between treatment should preferably be such that TSH is slightly elevated. This is in contrast to the suppressive dose of thyroxine, which should be instituted as soon as treatment is completed.

Radioiodine (^{131}I) is of use mainly in the treatment of metastatic disease, but it may also be used to treat the primary tumour when the condition is inoperable or when surgical removal has not been complete. The difficulty here, as mentioned previously, lies in distinguishing uptake in tumour from that in normal thyroid tissue. This problem may not be resolved until at least one ablative dose of ^{131}I has been given. Any subsequent uptake is likely to be located in tumour. External irradiation is usually advisable in addition to ^{131}I, even in those patients who do have a functioning primary tumour, because this ensures that all cells receive a radiation dose that is likely to destroy the tumour or at least render it incapable of further growth. Although the radiation dose from ^{131}I to some parts of a tumour may be very high, the variation in dose is such that some cells may escape serious damage.

For most patients, in particular those with bony metastases, ^{131}I therapy is unlikely to be curative, although some of these patients may survive for many years. There is no reason why external irradiation should not be used in combination with ^{131}I in patients with bony metastases, particularly if these are located in the vertebral column or in sites where a pathological fracture would result in a serious disability.

Some caution should be exercised in treating patients with pulmonary deposits, particularly when these are widespread, because radiation fibrosis may develop and eventually prove fatal (Rall et al. 1957; Silverberg et al. 1970).

It is difficult to assess the results of ^{131}I therapy in patients with metastatic disease, because patients with well-differentiated tumours may survive for a long time without any treatment at all. Results from Villejuif show a 5-year survival of 53% and a 10-year survival of 23% for patients with functioning metastases treated with ^{131}I (Tubiana et al. 1975). Patients with lung metastases, surprisingly, did better than those with bony metastases.

Role of Radiotherapy

Differentiated Thyroid Tumours

Surgery is the principal method of treatment for patients with differentiated thyroid carcinoma. For many patients, perhaps the majority, the disease is eradicated and no further treatment is required. It is difficult in this setting to evaluate the role of radiotherapy, the more so as the natural history of thyroid carcinoma is so variable and the progress of the disease is often very slow. Another factor that confuses the issue is that patients with differentiated tumours are usually maintained on thyroid hormone. This increases the difficulty of assessing any benefit from other methods of treatment, although there must be some uncertainty about the effectiveness of suppressive therapy in patients with tumours that do not necessarily behave in a uniform fashion. Even in large centres, experience in the management of patients with thyroid carcinoma is limited because the condition is rare and there is little opportunity for controlled trials or comparison of different methods of treatment. It would be helpful, for instance, to know whether ^{131}I given postoperatively was of value in patients without definite evidence of residual disease, but the answer to this sort of question could only be obtained by instituting national or international trials and following up patients for a very long time. In the absence of such information treatment policy cannot be too rigidly defined.

Undifferentiated Thyroid Tumours

It is usually possible to diagnose an undifferentiated thyroid tumour from the history and the clinical findings. Once this diagnosis is made a needle or drill biopsy should be performed, because patients with these tumours are best managed by radiotherapy, with or without chemotherapy, rather than by surgery.

The prognosis for patients with anaplastic tumours, in particular for those with tumours of the spindle- and giant-cell type, is poor. Most of them are dead within 6 months of starting treatment. There are, however, significant differences in the results of treatment if the various series reported in the literature are compared. In some series more than 20% of patients survived for 5 years, and these patients were probably cured of their disease (SMEDAL and MEISSNER 1961; RAFLA 1969). More recent reports on the treatment of patients with anaplastic spindle- and giant-cell tumours rarely show more than 5%–10% of patients surviving for more than 1 year (NISHIYAMA et al. 1972; KYRIAKIDES and SOSIN 1974; JEREB et al. 1975; ALDINGER et al. 1978). These discrepancies are probably due to lack of uniformity in the histological classification of thyroid tumours and to the inclusion of patients with small rouund-cell tumours in some series. THOMAS and BUCKWALTER (1973) found that the prognosis for patients with small round-cell tumours was very much better than that of patients with other types of anaplastic tumour, and that the behaviour and response of small round-cell tumours was similar to that of lymphoma.

It seems that spindle- and giant-cell tumours form a well-defined pathological entity with a uniformly bad prognosis. Other so-called anaplastic thyroid carcinomas probably include a variety of tumours, some of which are in fact lymphomas or at any rate behave like lymphomas. The distinction may be of more academic than practical importance.

Anaplastic Carcinoma

Anaplastic carcinomas are treated primarily by irradiation. These tumours are rarely amenable to surgery and it is doubtful whether anything is gained by an attempt to remove part of a tumour that is deemed to be inoperable. Survival data, however, suggest that the best results have been obtained in patients who were managed by a combination of surgery, radiotherapy, and chemotherapy (ALDINGER et al. 1978). It is clearly difficult to interpret this information, since the patients who were subjected to surgery presumably had less advanced disease, but there may well be a case for attempting thyroidectomy in patients who have tumours that are judged to be technically operable. In these patients, surgery should be regarded as a tumour-debulking procedure and should always be followed by radiotherapy, because the incidence of local recurrence is very high.

Radiotherapy should be started as soon as possible. If material for histological examination is obtained by drill or needle biopsy there need be no delay. In patients who present with symptoms of tracheal obstruction it is better to avoid a tracheostomy if possible, because this always interferes with and delays radiotherapy. The region treated should include the upper part of the mediastinum and the regional lymph nodes as well as the primary tumour. It may be advantageous to protract treatment and to aim at giving a dose of 6000 rads in 6 weeks, but it may not always be possible to achieve this dose.

Despite the poor prognosis, some patients are cured of this disease. Chemotherapy has been tried for anaplastic tumours, but the results so far have not been very encouraging. At Radiumhammet, methotrexate was found to prolong survival, but it produced severe complications and recurrence occurred as soon as treatment was discontinued (JEREB et al. 1975). Adriamycin, used either as a single agent (GOTTLIEB and STRATTON-HILL 1975) or in combination with vincristine and bleomycin (SOKAL and HARMER 1978), has had only limited success. Actinomycin D in combination with surgery and radiotherapy seemed to improve survival in one small series (ROGERS et al. 1974), but subsequent reports from the same centre were less enthusiastic. Nevertheless, in a condition that is so difficult to cure chemotherapy should probably be tried in selected cases.

Malignant Lymphoma

It may be very difficult to distinguish on histological grounds between an anaplastic carcinoma and a lymphoma (RAYFIELD et al. 1971). Certain features may help to clarify this diagnosis. A family history of thyroid disease, clinical or laboratory evidence of hypothyroidism, and the presence of thyroid autoantibodies would all favour pre-existing autoimmune thyroiditis, a condition known to be associated with thyroid lymphoma (WOOLNER et al. 1966; GOUDIE and ANGOURIDAKIS 1970; BURKE et al. 1977). The response to radiotherapy may also be helpful. Lymphomas usually show a quicker and more complete response than anaplastic carcinomas.

The prognosis for patients with thyroid lymphoma is much better than that of patients with undifferentiated carcinoma. Local recurrence after radiotherapy is exceptional. Although the condition is potentially curable, the results of treatment are not as good as one might expect with such a radiosensitive tumour.

WOOLNER et al. (1966) reviewed a series of 46 patients treated at the Mayo Clinic. In those who had invasive spread or lymph node involvement the outlook was not very good. Only eight of 30 patients (27%) were alive at the time of the follow-up survey. Patients treated by irradiation after undergoing biopsy seemed to fare rather better than those subjected to surgical resection followed by irradiation. For patients whose tumour was confined within the capsule of the thyroid the prognosis was good. Only one of the 16 patients in this group had died. A recent report from the MD Anderson Hospital gave similar conclusions with respect to the effect of local spread and regional lymph node involvement on survival (BURKE et al. 1977). Age was also important from the prognostic point of view. The overall 5-year survival rate was 54%, but for patients under the age of 65 it was 77%, whereas for those over the age of 65 it was 32%.

Treatment of thyroid lymphomas demands wide-field irraditation. The area treated should include both sides of the neck, extending as high as the tips of the mastoid processes, and inferiorly it should encompass at least the upper half of the mediastinum. Most of the supraclavicular and infraclavicular fossae should be included. Care should be taken to avoid exceeding the tolerance dose to the spinal cord. The technique is similar to that of mantle irradiation. The dose to the involved area should be 4000 rads in 4 weeks, but the dose to the mediastinum need not exceed 3500 rads provided there is no gross evidence of mediastinal disease.

The results of treatment for thyroid lymphoma could probably be improved by using chemotherapy in addition to radiotherapy. An appropriate drug combination is COP (cyclophosphamide, vincristine, and prednisolone) started a few weeks after radiotherapy has been completed, but if there is evidence of disseminated disease at the onset chemotherapy should precede radiotherapy.

Medullary Carcinoma

Medullary carcinoma of the thyroid (MCT) is best treated by surgery, a total thyroidectomy being carried out whenever possible. No further treatment is required if removal has been complete. Serum calcitonin should be measured before and after the operation. Raised levels after operation indicate either residual local disease or the presence of unsuspected metastases. If at operation it seems unlikely that the tumour can be completely resected it may nevertheless be advantageous to reduce its bulk by removing as much as possible and to follow this with radiotherapy, which should be given whenever there is any suspicion of residual tumour in the neck.

Information on the value of radiotherapy in the management of MCT is limited, but there seems to be a general impression that this tumour is totally unresponsive to irradiation. It has to be remembered that MCT is usually a very slow-growing tumour, and irradiation could not therefore be expected to result in any rapid shrinkage. Regression and sometimes complete resolution do occur after irradiation, however, albeit slowly, and several good responses to radiotherapy have been described in the literature (Halnan 1975; Tubiana et al. 1975; Harmer 1977).

References

1 Aldinger KA, Samaan NA, Ibanez M, Stratton-Hill C (1978) Anaplastic carcinoma of the thyroid. Cancer 41:2267

2 Burke JS, Butler JJ, Fuller LM (1977) Malignant lymphomas of the thyroid. Cancer 39:1587

3 Busnardo B, Vangelista R, Giarelli ME, Bui F, Lazzi C (1976) TSH levels and TSH response to TRH as a guide to the replacement treatment of patients with thyroid carcinoma. J Clin Endocrinol Metab 42:901

4 Catz B, Petit DW, Schwartz H, Davis F, McCammon C, Starr P (1959) Treatment of cancer of the thyroid postoperatively with suppressive thyroid medication, radioactive iodine, and thyroid-stimulating hormone. Cancer 12:371

5 Corbett BD, Cunningham RM, Halnan KE, Pochin EE (1956) A profile counter and its calibration. Phys Med Biol 1:37

6 Crile G (1968) Treatment of carcinomas of the thyroid. In: Young S, Inman DR (eds) Thyroid neoplasia. Academic Press, London New York, p 39

7 Einhorn J (1958) Studies on the effect of thyrotropic hormone on the thyroid function in man. Acta Radiol [Suppl] (Stockh) 160

8 Goolden AWG, Davey JB (1963) The ablation of normal thyroid tissue with iodine-131. Br J Radiol 36:340

9 Gottlieb JA, Stratton-Hill C (1975) Adriamycin (NSC-123127) therapy in thyroid carcinoma. Cancer Treat Rep 6:283

10 Goudie RB, Angouridakis CE (1970) Autoimmune thyroiditis associated with malignant lymphoma of the thyroid. J Clin Pathol 23:377

11 Halnan KE (1975) The non-surgical treatment of thyroid cancer. Br J Surg 62:769

12 Harmer CL (1977) External beam radiotherapy for thyroid cancer. Ann Radiol (Paris) 20:791

13 Hays MT, Solomon DH, Beall GN (1967) Suppression of human thyroid function by antibodies to bovine thyrotropin. J Clin Endocrinol Metab 27:1540

14 Hazard JB (1964) Thyroid neoplasia. In: Hazard JB, Smith DE (eds) The thyroid. Williams & Wilkins Baltimore (An international academy of pathology monograph, p 239)

15 Hazard JB, Hawk WA, Crile G (1959) Medullary (solid) carcinoma of the thyroid – a clinicopathological entity. J Clin Endocrinol Metab 19:152

16 Henk JM, Kirkman S, Owen GM (1972) Whole-body scanning and ^{131}I therapy in the management of thyroid carcinoma. Br J Radiol 45:369

17 Hershman JM, Edwards CL (1972) Serum thyrotropin (TSH) levels after thyroid ablation compared with TSH levels after exogenous bovine TSH: implications for ^{131}I treatment of thyroid carcinoma. J Clin Endocrinol Metab 34:815
18 Jereb B, Stjernsward J, Lowhagen T (1975) Anaplastic giant cell carcinoma of the thyroid: A study of treatment and prognosis. Cancer 35:1293
19 Kyriakides G, Sosin H (1974) Anaplastic carcinoma of the thyroid. Ann Surg 179:295
20 Nishiyama RH, Dunn EL, Thompson NW (1972) Anaplastic spindle cell and giant cell tumours of the thyroid. Cancer 30:113
21 Pochin EE (1967) Prospects from the treatment of thyroid carcinoma with radioiodine. Clin Radiol 18:113
22 Rafla S (1969) Anaplastic tumours of the thyroid. Cancer 23:668
23 Rall JE, Alpers JB, Lewallen CG, Sonenberg M, Berman M, Rawson RW (1957) Radiation pneumonitis and fibrosis: a complication of radioiodine treatment of pulmonary metastases from cancer of the thyroid. J Clin Endocrinol Metab 17:1263
24 Rayfield EJ, Nishiyama RH, Sisson JC (1971) Small cell tumours of the thyroid. Cancer 28:1023
25 Rogers JD, Lindberg RD, Hill CS, Gerhan EG (1974) Spindle and giant cell carcinoma of the thyroid. A different therapeutic approach. Cancer 34:1328
26 Russel WO, Ibanez ML, Clark RL, White EC (1963) Thyroid carcinoma. Classification, intraglandular dissemination and clinicopathological study based upon whole organ sections of 80 glands. Cancer 16:1425
27 Samaan NA, Beceiro JR, Stratton Hill C, Haynie TP, Glenn HJ (1972) Thyrotropin-releasing hormone (TRH) studies in patients with thyroid cancer. J Clin Endocrinol Metab 35:438
28 Scott JS, Halnan KE, Shimmins J, Kostaki P, Mackenzie H (1970) Measurement of dose to thyroid carcinoma metastases from radio-iodine therapy. Br J Radiol 43:256
29 Silverberg SG, Hutter RVP, Foster FW (1970) Fatal carcinoma of the thyroid. Histology, metastases and cause of death. Cancer 25:792
30 Smedal MI, Meissner WA (1961) The results of treatment in undifferentiated carcinoma of the thyroid. Radiology 76:927
31 Smedal MI, Salzman FA, Meissner WA (1967) The value of 2 MV roentgen-ray therapy in differentiated thyroid carcinoma. AJR 99:352
32 Smithers DW, Howard N, Trott NG (1965) Treatment of carcinoma of the thyroid with radioiodine. Br Med J 2:969
33 Sokal M, Harmer CL (1978) Chemotherapy for anaplastic carcinoma of the thyroid. Clin Oncol 4:3
34 Taunton OD, McDaniel HG, Pittman JA (1965) Standardization of TSH testing. J Clin Endocrinol Metab 25:266
35 Thomas CG, Buckwalter J (1973) Poorly differentiated neoplasms of the thyroid gland. Ann Surg 177:632
36 Tubiana M, Lacour J, Monnier JP, Bergiron C, Gerard-Marchant R, Roujeau J, Bok B, Parmentier C (1975) External radiotherapy and radioiodine in the treatment of 359 thyroid cancers. Br J Radiol 48:894
37 Varma VM, Beierwaltes WH, Nofal NM, Nishiyama RH, Copp JE (1970) Treatment of thyroid cancer. JAMA 214:1437
38 Woolner LB, Beahrs OH, Black BM, McConahey WM, Keating FR (1961) Classification and prognosis of thyroid carcinoma: a study of 885 observed cases in a thirty year period. Am J Surg 102:354
39 Woolner LB, McConahey WM, Beahrs OH, Black BM (1966) Primary malignant lymphoma of the thyroid. Am J Surg 111:502
40 Woolner LB, Beahrs OH, Black BM, McConahey WM, Keating FR (1969) Long-term survival rates. In: Hedinger CE (ed) Thyroid cancer. Springer, Berlin Heidelberg New York, p 326

Medical Management

J. A. Strong

Department of Medicine, University of Edinburgh and Western General Hospital,
GB-Edinburgh EH4 2XU

Introduction

Generalizations about the treatment of disease, as in so many matters, involve inherent dangers. Few would disagree, however, that when cancer of the thyroid gland has been diagnosed, the treatment, when this is possible, should be surgical in nature, supported by irradiation. This in turn can be given from external sources or, when feasible, as radioiodine. Medical management might be taken to cover the whole train of events from the time when the patient first comes under observation, but for present purposes it will be restricted to the measures available when surgery and irradiation have nothing further to offer. The need for a critical eye and a sensitive ear for changes in signs and symptoms, for early evidence of complications, and for the need to adjust treatment in response to changing requirements must be emphasized.

The responsibility for monitoring the progress of this group of patients should lie with a clinical organization equipped to recognize relevant changes and to use to advantage the extending range of laboratory technology now available. Thyroid function and treatment can be controlled with a new dimension of precision since reliable assays have become available, e.g., for thyroxine (T_4), triiodothyronine (T_3), thyroid-stimulating hormone (TSH), and now also for thyroglobulin (TG). Scanning techniques can be used to advantage to demarcate the extent and activity of disease, and drugs are available to control the function of thyroid tissue. The range of chemotherapeutic agents has been extended more rapidly than they can be assessed for their value in the management of thyroid cancer. There is therefore all the more need, when dealing with a relatively uncommon form of cancer, for a method of pooling information and of planning chemotherapeutic trials in such a way that valid conclusions on the efficacy of these drugs can be reached, so that their worth is not overlooked and, on the other hand, they do not gain an unjustified credibility.

For present purposes, the following four aspects of medical management will be discussed: continuing surveillance, replacement therapy with thyroid hormones, tumour-suppressive therapy, and finally cytotoxic chemotherapy. Early diagnosis and preventive aspects of the problem, although highly relevant, will not be considered further.

Continuing Surveillance

Surveillance is attended by the danger common to so many long-term problems, that division of responsibility between so many may mean indifferent management overall. The family doctor who sees the patient first and often last, the surgeon who operates, the physician or endocrinologist, the laboratory services, the radiotherapist or nuclear medicine expert with medical physicist support, and sometimes the oncologist with chemotherapy to offer all have a contribution to make to the study and the care of patients with thyroid cancer. Different solutions have been developed to meet the difficulties, including joint clinics between the interested groups, but these are extravagant of professional time. They have the major virtue of concentrating experience, however, and should make it easier to organize effective therapeutic trials. A series of visits to a range of clinics may otherwise be imposed, which cannot be other than a test of tolerance for the individual patient. We have had experience with the long-term surveillance of other forms of thyroid disease, and have devised a method that could easily be adapted to the care of thyroid cancer, namely the Scottish Automated Follow-up Register (SAFUR), which at least provides a method of maintaining continuity of care (Hedley et al. 1970) and ensuring that the patient and the doctors concerned are alerted to the need for a prearranged review.

Replacement and Suppressive Therapy

In the normal course of treatment of thyroid carcinoma, thyroidectomy or subtotal thyroidectomy will be performed in many cases. It is unlikely that the need for replacement therapy in these circumstances will be overlooked, though there may be a need for care in deciding what dose to use, whether T_4 or T_3 is more appropriate, when to initiate treatment, and whether to provide cover with a β-adrenergic receptor blocker, e.g., propranolol. The need for this precaution is found mainly in patients starting treatment who may have been clinically hypothyroid or even myxoedematous. If they are known to have angina pectoris or other evidence of ischaemic heart disease, they must certainly be given cover with a β-blocker, at least until they have adjusted to an effective level of replacement therapy, when the β-blocker might be cautiously withdrawn. Propranolol is the preparation preferred for this purpose, usually in doses of 20 mg every 8 h.

The concept of hormone dependence has been familiar for many years, particularly with hormone therapy of breast cancer. In the case of the thyroid gland, suppression of secretion of the supporting hormone, namely pituitary TSH, by the administration of thyroid hormone was advocated by Dunhill (1937) more than 40 years ago. Balme (1954) described a single case with pulmonary metastases that disappeared when T_4 was given, and Crile (1970) has repeatedly emphasized the value of suppressive treatment with thyroid hormone. The object must be to suppress secretion of TSH, and in the normal course of events this can be achieved with about 0.2 mg T_4 or up to 100 μg T_3 daily. The only virtue of T_3 over T_4 is the speed with which its suppressive effect disappears when the treatment is withdrawn, and this has obvious advantages when serial treatment with ^{131}I is being given to a patient with a tumour capable of concentrating ^{131}I.

The relationship between the hypothalamic hormone TRH, the pituitary hormone TSH, and the thyroid hormones T_4 and T_3 has been described in Chap. 4. We can activate or block the system in various ways. So far as thyroid cancer is concerned, the suggestion that prolonged and persistent stimulation of the thyroid gland by TSH is a factor in promoting neoplastic change in the gland remains. There is much experimental evidence, reviewed by Doniach in 1974, to suggest that such a relationship exists in animals, but to be effective the stimulation must continue for half their lifespan or more. There is some clinical evidence in man also to support this concept. The remedy is simple and relatively innocuous, and the need can be recognized by a single plasma TSH assay.

Replacement and suppressive therapy are therefore coincidental, and in the usual case of thyroid cancer, T_4 should be given in sufficient doses to maintain suppression of TSH production. This amount will vary between 0.15 and 0.3 mg per day in different individuals, and successful suppression can of course be confirmed by TSH assay, a procedure that is now readily available. The TRH test described by HALL et al. (1974) can be added to ensure that treatment is adequate not only to keep the blood level of TSH low, but to suppress it to the point where no response or a minimal response is elicited when TRH is given. This, however, seems scarcely necessary since it may involve giving doses of T_4 that are sufficiently large to make the patient mildly thyrotoxic (CREUTZIG et al. 1977; LAMBERG et al. 1977).

Before leaving the subject of replacement therapy, it should be recalled that during the course of thyroid ablation, the parathyroid glands may also be destroyed. Parathyroid hormone cannot be used as replacement therapy and an analogue of vitamin D is usually employed for this purpose. Calciferol 1.25 mg once daily, or preferably dihydrotachysterol 0.2 mg once daily is a satisfactory starting point, but the dose required to maintain a normal serum calcium and inorganic phosphate concentration varies widely between individuals and indeed may do so with time in the same individual, so that when using these agents it is essential to check the serum calcium level at intervals of no more than 1 month at first, and when stability has been achieved, at intervals of approximately 3 months. It may be that in future the newer analogue of vitamin D, 1-α-hydroxy vitamin D3 (alfacalcidol), in doses of 1 μg daily, or the active metabolite of vitamin D, 1,25,dihydroxy vitamin D3 (calcitriol), in a daily dose of 0.25 μg will be more satisfactory. At present they are many times more expensive than calciferol, and their advantage has not yet been confirmed, except that when overdosage does occur with alfacalcidol the withdrawal of treatment is followed by a faster return to normal than with calciferol.

Cytotoxic Chemotherapy

In the past 5 years a number of reports have appeared on the use of chemotherapeutic agents for the treatment of progressive thyroid carcinoma that was not controlled by other, more conventional methods. In general, these reports deal with relatively small groups of patients with a wide range of ages; they include a variety of histological types of tumour (though in the main anaplastic); controls are not employed; and the definition of a favourable response is often one of very marginal benefit. In some cases several drugs have been used in the same trial, sometimes a combination of drugs in the same patient, and somewhat arbitrary doses. Chemotherapy may have been given before entry to the trial. Thus the conditions under which this form of therapy has been used are most unfavourable. The problem is compounded by the relative scarcity of patients who would be selected for participation in treatment schedules of this type, and this state of affairs is likely to continue until comprehensive collaborative clinical trials can be organized or until there is a major improvement in the efficacy of the chemotherapy available.

GOTTLIEB and HILL (1974) reported on the use of doxorubicin (adriamycin) in 30 patients treated after surgery, radiotherapy, and radioiodine had been exploited to the full. Eleven patients showed a partial remission: all histological types of tumour were involved, and the median duration of response was 7 months (range 2 to more than 38 months). Three of five cases of medullary carcinoma of the thyroid responded. The dose of doxorubicin used was restricted mainly by the incidence of cardiomyopathy, and also by a number of other, less serious side effects.

Table 1. Data obtained in trials of chemotherapy in thyroid cancer

Authors	Drug used	No. of patients reported	Remission rate (%)
GOTTLIEB and HILL (1974)	Doxorubicin (adriamycin)	30	37
RICCABONA et al. (1976)	Combination of: 6-mercaptopurine, procarbazine, cyclophosphamide, 5-fluorouracil, amethopterine, vinblastine, 6-methylprednisolone	44	Not specified
SHIMAOKA and REYES (1976)	Doxorubicin Bleomycin *cis*-DDP Podophyllotoxin Cyclophosphamide Other drugs Combinations of above	25	40
BENKER et al. (1977)	Combined doxorubicin and bleomycin	21	38
ROSENCWEIG (1977)	*cis*-DDP	Not specified	"Promising"
SOKAL and HARMER (1978)	Combined doxorubicin, vincristine, bleomycin	14	64

Doxorubicin has featured as the drug most commonly used in several of the other trials reported, but in none has a more favourable conclusion emerged than that provided by GOTTLIEB and HILL (1974).

ROSENCWEIG et al. (1977) have recently described the use of *cis*-platinum (*cis*-diamminedichloroplatinum: DDP in a variety of malignant tumours, including some arising in the thyroid gland. Other authors have also mentioned the use of this drug, which is generally described as promising.

Since the benefits to be derived from the use of these drugs is so marginal, their use can still only be recommended in circumstances where more conventional methods have failed, where pain is a prominent feature, where the therapist responsible already has experience in the use of these drugs, and, preferably, where the outcome can be used in comparative assessments with larger groups of patients.

The data available from a number of trials are summarized in Table 1. On the basis of these and other data, HALNAN (1977) has provided a therapeutic regimen that might follow conventional methods when indicated, but probably only for anaplastic tumours and lymphomas. This combines doxorubicin, cyclophosphamide, 5-fluorouracil, and vincristine. For elderly debilitated patients he advises a combination of chlorambucil and prednisolone.

Conclusions

Replacement therapy and suppressive therapy in thyroid cancer are important simple measures that influence the patients' general welfare and perhaps the behaviour of the tumour. Advantage should be taken of the facilities now available to monitor the efficacy of therapy given in this way.

The disease is relatively so uncommon that experience gained in the chemotherapy of thyroid cancer should be pooled, so far as possible, but this would mean the acceptance of common therapeutic protocols. The benefits of chemotherapy are still so marginal at present that careful discrimination is essential in the application of this form of treatment.

References

1 Balme HW (1954) Metastatic carcinoma of the thyroid successfully treated with thyroxine. Lancet 1:812–813
2 Benker G, Hackenberg K, Hoff HG, Seeber S, Elke J, Windeck R, Reinwein D (1977) Combined doxorubicin and bleomycin treatment of metastasising thyroid carcinoma: results in 21 patients. Dtsch Med Wochenschr 102:1908–1913
3 Creutzig H, Kallfelz I, Haindl H, Schulle R, Hundeshagen H (1977) Hormone replacement in patients with carcinoma of the thyroid. Dtsch Med Wochenschr 102:1763–1766
4 Crile G (1970) The endocrine dependency of papillary carcinomas of the thyroid. In: Smithers DW (ed) Tumours of the thyroid gland. Livingstone, Edinburgh, pp 269–275
5 Doniach I (1974) Experimental evidence of etiology of thyroid cancer. Proc R Soc Med 67:1103
6 Dunhill T (1937) The Lettsomian Lectures. The surgery of the thyroid gland. Trans Med Soc Lond 60:234
7 Gottlieb JA, Hill CS (1974) Chemotherapy of thyroid cancer with adriamycin: experience with 30 patients. N Engl J Med 290:193–197
8 Hall R, Anderson J, Smart GA, Besser M (1974) Fundamentals of clinical endocrinology, 2nd edn. Pitman Medical, London, pp 81–82
9 Halnan KE (1977) The treatment of thyroid cancer. Ann Radiol 20:826–830
10 Hedley AJ, Scott AM, Weir RD, Crooks J (1970) Computer-assisted follow-up register for the North-east of Scotland. Br Med J 1:556–558
11 Lamberg BA, Rantanen M, Saarinen P (1977) Choosing thyroxine dose after treatment of thyroid cancer. Lancet 2:1290–1291
12 Riccabona G, Zechmann W, Fill H (1975) Cytostatic drug therapy of thyroid cancer. In: Robbins J (ed) Thyroid research. Excerpta Medica, Amsterdam, pp 583–585
13 Rosencweig M, von Hoff DD, Slavik M, Muggia FM (1977) Cis-diamminedichloroplatinum. A new anti-cancer drug. Ann Intern Med 86:803–812
14 Shimaoka K, Reyes J (1975) Chemotherapy of thyroid carcinoma. In: Robbins J (ed) Thyroid research. Excerpta Medica, Amsterdam, pp 586–589
15 Sokal M, Harmer CL (1978) Chemotherapy for anaplastic carcinoma of the thyroid. Clin Oncol 4:3–10

Perspectives and Prospects

K. E. Halnan

Department of Radiotherapy and Oncology, Royal Postgraduate Medical School
and Hammersmith Hospital, GB-London W12 OHS

Introduction

The aspects of thyroid cancer covered in this volume need to be put into perspective within the context of clinical oncology and cancer as a whole.

It may be considered that thyroid cancer is of little importance in oncology. Certainly thyroid cancer is rare. It may also be suggested that in the main it presents in two categories: well-differentiated tumours, which run an inherently benign course requiring only minimal conservative treatment, and undifferentiated tumours associated with a very poor prognosis whatever treatment is given. Despite its rarity, thyroid cancer is highly relevant to oncology in general, and its study repays considerable time and effort. If it were possible to cure all types of thyroid cancer, our knowledge would obviously be adequate to allow us to cure all types of cancer at other sites.

Prognosis

Prognosis is central to the whole problem. Adequate knowledge has usually been bedevilled in the past by small numbers and by the processes of selection involved in referral and in allocation to treatment. Conversely the large series reported from cancer registration schemes, and the large bodies of regional, national, and international data, may be unreliable because of considerable variability in the quality, nomenclature, and criteria of histological diagnosis.

Very good data are now becoming available from the Thyroid Cooperative Group of the European Organisation for Research on Treatment of Cancer (EORTC). The histological reviews have been performed by a distinguished group of pathologists, including Dilwyn Williams, who has also contributed to this volume, and the registration, analysis, and statistics have come under the care of Richard Sylvester in the EORTC data centre in Brussels. About 1400 or more cases have been registered and the following discussion refers to 591 of these with actuarial survival data. Good statistics are available to demonstrate the importance of age, sex, histology, and extent of primary and secondary tumour (by TNM staging), and these have enabled Sylvester to construct a Prognostic Index of remarkable reliability.

The importance of age at diagnosis and of sex has been amply confirmed. It is apparent (Fig. 1) that there is a steady fall in survival with increasing age of the patient at diagnosis, from the 6-year survival of over 90% in children and young adults under 35, through the 35–44 group (85% alive at 6 years), the 45–54 group (65%), and the 55–64 group (55%),

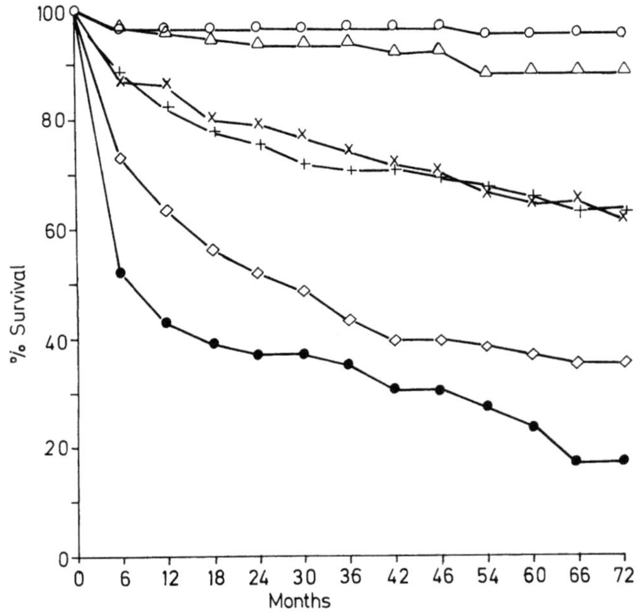

Fig. 1. Actuarial survival curve for thyroid cancer, by age at diagnosis. Figures in parentheses show numbers of patients. ⊙, < 31 (110); △, 31–40 (90); +, 41–50 (99); ×, 51–60 (104); ◈, 61–70 (133); ↑, 71 and over (55). BYAR et al. (to be published)

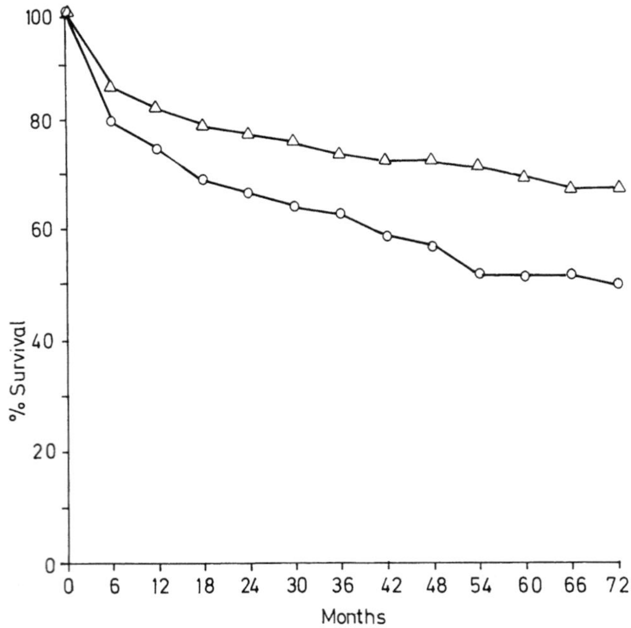

Fig. 2. Actuarial survival curve for thyroid cancer, by sex. ⊙, male patients (190); △, female (401). BYAR et al. (to be published)

down to the over 65 s, only a quarter of whom survive for 6 years. Women survive conspicuously better in all age groups, with an overall 6-year survival of about 67%, compared with only about 50% of men (Fig. 2).

Histological classification has been analyzed in two ways, by principal cell type and by main associated cell type, as described already by WILLIAMS (Chap. 5, this volume). The sensible

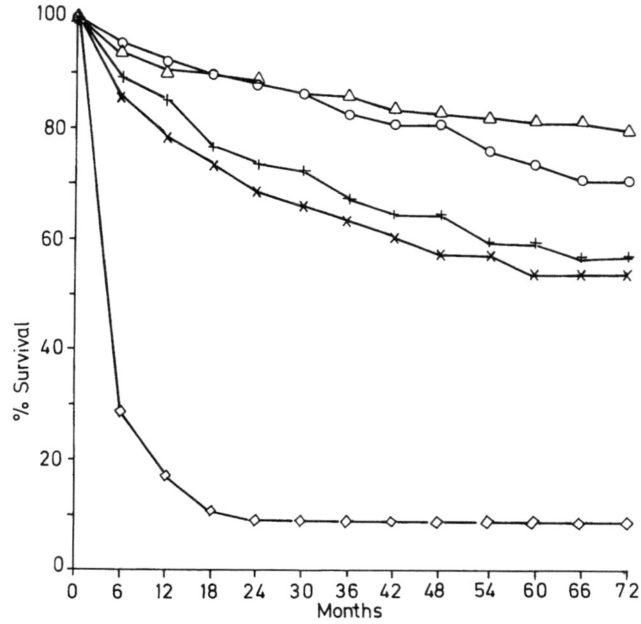

Fig. 3. Actuarial survival curve for thyroid cancer, by principal cell type. ⊙, follicular, well differentiated (131); +, follicular, less well differentiated (106); ◈, anaplastic (77); △, papillary (227); ×, medullary (43). BYAR et al. (to be published)

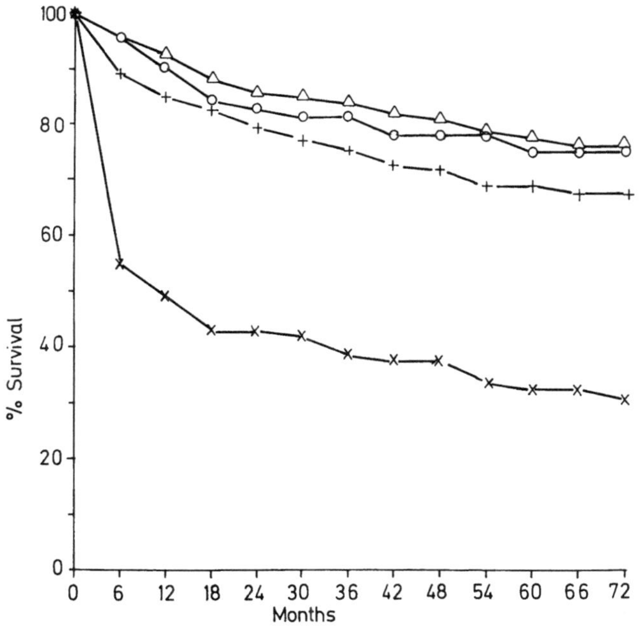

Fig. 4. Actuarial survival curve for thyroid cancer by extent (UICC TNM classification) of primary tumour. ⊙, T0 (71); △, T1 (126); +, T2 (212); ×, T3 (110). BYAR et al. (to be published)

classification is of papillary, follicular, medullary, and anaplastic carcinoma, with a very useful division of the follicular group into well and less well differentiated. It can be seen that anaplastic cancer patients do poorly, but nevertheless over 10% can achieve over 5-year survival, and also that there are apparently two groups with similar survival rates – papillary and well-differentiated follicular cancer and medullary and poorly differentiated follicular cancer

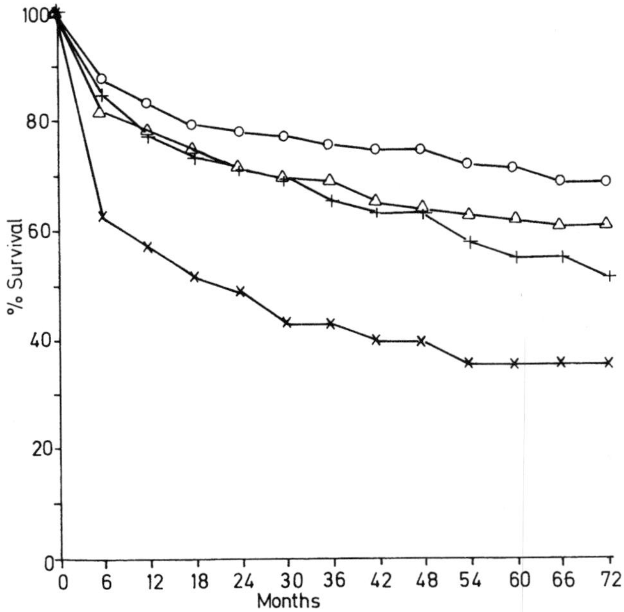

Fig. 5. Actuarial survival curve for thyroid cancer, by clinical evaluation (UICC TNM classification) of regional lymph nodes. ⊙, N0 (290); △, N1 (163); +, N2 (55); ×, N3 (38). BYAR et al. (to be published)

(Fig. 3). Knowledge of the importance of associated cells is even more interesting, confirming suspicions that the presence of anaplastic cells in a well-differentiated tumour implies just as bad a prognosis as if the whole cancer were anaplastic, i.e., that the prognosis is that of the worst type of cell present in the tumour, whether it be in the minority or majority.

The extent or stage of the tumour has been shown to be of prognostic significance: the TNM system *is* of value. It seems, however, that it is only necessary to know the stage of the *primary* tumour for the prognosis to be inferred, and that there are only two prognostic groups when the patients are divided according to the stage of their primary tumour: survival is similar with stages T 0, T 1, and T 2, but a T 3 tumour (i.e., one that has invaded the capsule) certainly has a significantly worse outlook (Fig. 4).

It is often said, especially by our American colleagues, that involvement of lymph nodes, and knowledge of their status, is of little prognostic value in thyroid cancer. European patients, however, are seen to survive progressively less well with increasing extent of node involvement from N 0 to N 3 (Fig. 5).

The presence of distant metastases should obviously be expected to, and in fact does, make prognosis substantially worse. An interesting new point, however, is that the presence of only a *single* metastatis at diagnosis entails a prognosis intermediate between that of no metastases and that of multiple metastases.

SYLVESTER has constructed (mathematically) a prognostic index with risk groups related to survival (Tables 1 and 2).

This may seem complex, but in fact it simply applies mathematical weighting to the observed importance for prognosis of all the different relevant factors. Observed survival rates are found to be remarkably similar to the values on the survival curves predicted from this formula.

The main clinical message to be conveyed is not only that age, sex, histology, and stage are all important, but that they must be clearly stated and their importance remembered when the

Table 1. Proposed EORTC prognostic index for thyroid carcinoma

Age at diagnosis (in years)
+ 12 if male
+ 10 if medullary or if principal cell type is follicular and less differentiated, provided that the associated cell type is not anaplastic
+ 45 if principal or associated cell type is anaplastic
+ 10 if T category is T 3
+ 15 if there is at least one distant metastatic site
+ 15 *in addition to above* if there are multiple distant metastatic sites
= Total score

Table 2. Risk groups, based on total scores with observed survival rates

Total score	Risk group	5-Year actuarial survival (%)
< 50	1	95
50– 65	2	80
66– 83	3	51
84–108	4	33
≥ 109	5	5

Table 3. Good prognostic group – all these criteria must be fullfilled

Under 35 years of age
Tumour T 1 or T 2 (i.e., not invading thyroid capsule)
No metastases
Papillary or follicular; well-differentiated histology

value of treatment is assessed. On the question as to whether treatment is needed at all, surely the demonstrable answer is that the only group with a really good prognosis (90% survival at 5 years) is the one satisfying all the criteria listed in Table 3.

In this group it is necessary to think seriously about long-term hazards from radical surgery, X-ray therapy, and chemotherapy – and to consider each individual patient very carefully indeed. Social and other factors, such as the ability of the patient to come for close follow-up visits and the place of the patient's home, will also be relevant. There will be some patients in this group, and *only* in this group, for whom no more treatment than surgery and hormone therapy (thyroxine) will be advisable, together with a good follow-up system.

Table 4. Calcitonin: tumour marker for MTC

Measurable by radioimmunoassay
Normal levels less than 0.10 ng/ml
Highly specific for medullary thyroid cancer except for slightly raised levels in a few other tumours, especially small-cell bronchial cancer and breast cancer
Doubtful levels can be checked by alcohol or calcium provocation (COOMBES et al., 1974)

Control

It has been shown that the prognosis of most other cases of thyroid cancer is indeed such that the best treatment is needed, so that the question of management must be considered. According to the modern approach, cancer management begins with very careful investigation or staging. This should include all the relevant investigations, in particular not only radioiodine scanning but also a bone scan, full investigation of thyroid function, and full radiological screening, preferably by computerized tomography. One of the most important investigations, when relevant, is the assay of index substances or tumour markers in the serum, and fortunately there are now at least two good ones to consider.

Medullary Carcinoma

Medullary thyroid cancer (MCT) is a tumour that should now be capable of complete control. The main key to this is its own highly specific and sensitive marker substance – calcitonin. This marker is almost too easily measurable, since we are already often in the position, e.g., after total thyroidectomy, of finding raised or abnormal levels and being unable to detect residual, recurrent, or metastatic tumour cells by any other means, physical examination, radiology of chest and bones, (perhaps) CT scanning, (perhaps) lymphography, and liver scanning and function all yielding normal results (Table 4).

Calcitonin measurement may also be used to screen relatives of affected patients, and preventive or curative treatment can then be achieved. This has recently been well demonstrated in one family – the J. kindred – investigated at Tufts University, Boston, USA (GRAZE et al. 1978). Eighty-three of the 107 family members have been studied; 12 patients with carcinoma were found before 1970. Initial screening in 1970–1971 revealed 12 more patients with raised calcitonin, all of whom had carcinoma. Between 1971 and 1978 a further 21 patients were found to have raised calcitonin levels, and these have undergone thyroidectomy – 13 had no more than C-cell hyperplasia and 8 had early carcinoma (mean diameter only 0.2 cm) with no lymph node metastases. Measurement of carcinoembryonic antigen (CEA) is also of value (DELELLIS et al. 1978). This is a very worthwhile achievement in this rare tumour, but calcitonin measurement will accordingly only be relevant in about 7% of all thyroid cancers, which are themselves uncommon.

Well-Differentiated Carcinoma

Serum marker for differentiated cancer is now also available, namely thyroglobulin. It has been shown by VAN HERLE and UFFER (1975) that sensitive and consistent measurement of thyroglobulin is possible by means of radioimmunoassay and that the normal concentration in serum is less than 21 ng/ml. Elevated serum thyroglobulin levels can be found in patients with benign adenomas as well as those with differentiated carcinoma, so that there is little value in the measurement until after thyroidectomy, but it is a good and clear indication of the presence and extent of metastases and their response to treatment. Serum thyroglobulin is apparently not secreted by undifferentiated carcinomas or by MCT. This subject deserves attention in other laboratories, and some current work has been described in Chap. 8 by MAISEY and NG TANG FUI. Studies are also in progress in Glasgow and in Paris.

Management

This interesting work with tumour markers clearly can only be of value, practically or academically, if the metastases detected can be successfully treated and if multiple metastases are present a systemic treatment will have to be used, most probably chemotherapy, less probably immunotherapy.

Thyroid cancer continues to be so uncommon that information about its response to chemotherapy remains scanty and meagre. It is at least clear that it is unfortunately beyond question that its sensitivity to chemotherapy is no greater than that of other adenocarcinomas and undifferentiated tumours. There is good evidence that adriamycin (doxorubicin) can be of value, and suggestions that bleomycin, epipodophyllotoxin (VP 16-213), and *cis*-platinum (DDP) can also be effective. Cyclophosphamide, vincristine and vinblastine, 5-fluorouracil, the nitrosoureas, and methotrexate would seem to justify careful trial.

One current need is to find good combinations of drugs that are effective against advanced disease, which might then be used against microscopic metastases. Too few trials are going on; the EORTC group are active and there is at least one active trial in the United States (DURIE et al. 1979).

Conventional management by surgery and by radiotherapy remains of considerable importance and value, as has been emphasized throughout this volume. Surgery is still recommended for apparently benign nodular goitres – this is the best way of ensuring early detection, and possible surgical cure, of many unsuspected thyroid cancers. Surely one successful cancer cure by thyroidectomy will justify 50 thyroidectomies for benign lesions? No surgeon hesitates to biopsy or excise undiagnosed breast lumps. Appropriate and adequate radiotherapy with megavoltage X-rays or high-energy electrons, and with radioiodine, needs to be given – X-ray therapy is often of much more value than is commonly suggested. Hormone treatment is indubitably of value but cannot be relied on for ever; the only trial of its sole use known to the present author was abandoned because tumours escaped control and needed other treatment (THOMAS and BURNS 1961).

Malignant Lymphoma

Thyroid lymphoma is a subdivision that needs clearer identification; it seems common in Western Scotland, it occurs in elderly patients, and it can spread to the gastrointestinal tract. It needs as careful assessment and treatment by radiation and chemotherapy as does any other lymphoma; the main difficulty is the differential diagnosis from small-cell undifferentiated carcinoma.

Table 5. Situations involving same risk (1 in 10^6) of death

400 miles air travel
60 miles car travel in UK
Smoking $^3/_4$ of a cigarette
$1^1/_2$ weeks' factory work
20 min life as a man aged 60 years
0.5 rad to the thyroid causing cancer

Prevention

Prevention should not be neglected. It is still not known whether the simple inexpensive addition of iodide to salt could help in the prevention of cancer. Evidence on the association of endemic goitre, low iodine diet, and cancer seems contradictory. A fresh attempt is needed.

Finally, one definite aetiological agent, ionizing radiation, really needs to be put in perspective, since the death rate from radiation-induced thyroid cancer is very low. Pochin (1978) has shown how this can be done for radiation protection (Table 5), and the risk from radiation-induced thyroid cancer has also been indicated.

Conclusions

Thyroid cancer is uncommon and repays very careful study and management; it consists of at least five main subgroups, each needing different management by integrated combined treatment (Halnan 1980). Good histology is the key to good management, combined with full staging before treatment.

Prognosis can now be predicted accurately.

Three tumour markers, thyroglobulin, calcitonin, and CEA, need further study.

Treatment with appropriate combinations of surgery, radiotherapy, and hormones is necessary and worthwhile; chemotherapy needs much more investigation. A new approach to prevention and aetiology is needed.

References

1 Byar DP, Green SB, Dor P, Williams ED, Cohen J, van Gilse HA, Sylvester RJ, van Glabbeke M (to be published) A prognostic index for thyroid carcinoma – an EORTC study. Eur J Cancer

2 Coombes RC, Hillyard C, Greenberg PB, MacIntyre I (1974) Plasma-immunoreactive-calcitonin in patients with non-thyroid tumours. Lancet 1:1080–1083

3 DeLellis RA, Wolfe HJ, Rule AH, Reichlin S, Tashjian AH (1978) C.E.A. as a tissue marker in medullary thyroid carcinoma. N Engl J Med 299:1082

4 Durie B, Hellman D, Woolfenden J, Kartchmer M, O'Mara R, Salmon S (1979) Adjuvant therapy of thyroid cancer. In: Salmon SE, Jones SE (eds) Adjuvant therapy of cancer II. Grune & Stratton, New York, pp 198–204

5 Graze K, Spiler IJ, Tashjian AH, Melvin KEW, Cervi-Skinner S, Gager RF, Miller HH, Wolfe HJ, DeLellis RA, Leape L, Feldman ZT, Reichlin S (1978) Natural history of familial thyroid cancer. N Engl J Med 299:980–985
6 Halnan KE (1980) Treatment of thyroid cancer. In: Halnan KE (ed) Cancer treatment. Chapman & Hall, London, chapter 14
7 Pochin EE (1978) Why be quantitative about radiation risk estimates? Lauriston S. Taylor lectures in radiation protection and measurements. Lecture No. 2. National council on radiation protection and measurements. Washington D.C. 20014, USA
8 Thomas CG, Burns SD (1961) Studies on the dependency of thyroid cancer. In: Pitt-Rivers R (ed) Advances in thyroid research. Pergamon, London, p 350
9 Van Herle AJ, Uller RP (1975) Elevated serum thyroglobulin, a marker of metastases in differentiated thyroid carcinoma. J Clin Invest 56:272–277

Subject Index

actinomycin-D 120
adenoma 31
– and arrhemoblastoma 50
adriamycin 120, 127
aetiology 8f.
age, incidence 23, 104
–, specific mortality rates 1
–,– survival rates 129
Ailingnae Islanders 26
alfacalcidol 126
amethopterine 127
anaplastic carcinoma 8, 32, 50, 103, 106
– –, management 108, 120, 126
angiography 89
angio-invasive carcinoma 108, 112, 115
antibodies, microsomal 56, 57
–, thyroglobulin 56, 57
–, thyroid stimulating 58
atomic bomb explosions, Japan 15, 26
– – –, Pacific islands 25
auto-immune thyroiditis 9, 35, 52, 56
automated follow-up register 125

biochemical markers, calcitonin 60
– –, carcino-embryonic antigen 65
– –, histaminase 65
– –, thyroglobulin 73, 82, 134
biopsy, needle 73, 108, 119
bleomycin 120, 135
bone metastases 93
– scan 43

^{131}caesium scan 73
calciferol 126
calcification in thyroid tumors 89
calcitonin in familial medullary cancer 62, 134
– in management 62, 122, 134
– in non-thyroid tumors 61
–, provocative tests 63
– in sporadic medullary cancer 60
calcitrol 126
carcino-embryonic antigen 65, 134
causation 10f.
C-cells 47
–, hyperplasia 62, 134
–, neoplasia 47, 62
cervical lymph node metastases 49, 106, 120
childhood cancers 8, 23, 129
chlorambucil 127
cholecystokinin 65
chronic thyroiditis 9, 49
clinical presentation 68, 104
cold nodule 37, 70, 75, 87, 107, 110
computerised tomography 73, 98
control of thyroid function 37
– – growth 37
Cowden's syndrome 50
cyclophosphamide 127, 135
cytoxic chemotherapy 120f.

developmental anomalies 31
differentiated carcinoma, age incidence 102
– –, management 74, 113, 119
– – pathology 47
– –, prognosis 24, 130
dihydrotachysterol 126
doxorubicin, see adriamycin
dysphagia 105

epidemiology 1
–, international statistics 4
–, routine statistics 6
epipodophyllotoxin 135

familial studies 8, 62, 134
– syndromes 8
fibrosarcoma 109
fluorescent excitation analysis 73
– scanning 38
fluorouracil 127, 135
follicular carcinoma, incidence 26, 32, 104
– –, management 107, 114, 115
– –, pathology 47, 50
– –, results 108, 115, 131

^{67}gallium scan 73
Gardner's syndrome 50, 97
genetic factors 8, 50
giant-cell tumors 120
goitre and cancer 7, 9, 49
– –, histology 24
– –, nodular 9, 32, 71
– –, simple 32, 49
Grave's disease and cancer 57
– ophthalmopathy 58

haemangio-endothelioma 51
Hashimoto's thyroiditis 9, 35, 52, 56
Hiroshima 15
histaminase 65
histological classification 47f.
hoarseness 106
Hodgkin's disease 48
hormone dependence 114, 125
– –, childhood tumors 110
– –, differentiated carcinomas 113
– –, papillary carcinomas 114
– –, undifferentiated carcinomas 108
hot nodule 69
hyperparathyroidism, elevated calcitonin 61
hyperthyroidism and thyroid cancer 9, 13, 29, 33, 57
hypocalcaemia 107
hypoparathyroidism 126

incidence 1f., 23
–, latent thyroid cancer 7
^{123}iodine 69, 70
^{125}iodine 69
^{131}iodine in treatment 42, 108, 116
– in scans 69f.
iodine, dietary 32, 50
–, protein bound 41
iodine-plasma inorganic 42
irradiation hazards, atomic explosions 15, 24
– –, cervical adenitis 11, 49
– – in childhood 11, 28
– –, diagnostic radiology 16, 49
– –, hyperthyroidism 13
– –, lymphomas 11, 49
– –, minimising risk 13, 134
– –, risk estimates 25, 136
– –, therapeutic radiation 10f.
– –, thymic enlargement 11, 28, 49
– –, tinea capitis 28, 49
– –, use of radio-iodine 14, 29

latent period 24
– thyroid cancer 7
LATS 34, 58
LATS-P 34, 58
lingual thyroid 32
– – cancer 88
lung metastases 93
– –, CT scanning 99
lymph node metastases, cervical 90
– – –, mediastinal 90, 97
lymphoma malignant, auto-immune disease 35
– –, chemotherapy 121
– –, management 121, 135
– –, pathology 52

management 113
–, cytotoxic drugs 120, 126
–, radio-iodine 108
–, radiotherapy 115
–, surgery 107
–, thyroxine 107, 110, 125
–, tri-iodothyronine 125
Marshall Islanders 25, 29
mediastinal lymph node metastases 90, 97
medullary carcinoma, biochemical markers 62, 63, 122, 134
– –, familial 8, 62, 97, 134
– –, management 109, 122
– –, nephrocalcinosis 97
– –, pathology 51
– –, results 109
– –, screening 134

– –, sporadic 60, 97
mercaptopurine 127
metastases from thyroid cancer, liver 80
– – –, lymph node 49
– – –, pattern of spread 106
– – –, pulmonary 80
– – –, site distribution 90
metastatic tumors in thyroid 35, 109
mortality rates 3f.
– –, age specific 1
– –, histological types 7
– –, occupational 3, 16
– –, social class 4
multiple endocrine adenomatosis 62

Nagasaki 15
nephrocalcinosis 97
neutron irradiation hazards 27, 29
nitrosoureas 135
nodular goitre 9, 32
nuclear incidence 68

ophthalmopathy and thyroid cancer 58
ovarian tumours and thyroid cancer 50

papillary carcinoma, causation 10, 26, 32
– –, incidence 102, 104
– –, management 107, 113
– –, pathology 47, 48
– –, results 114, 131
para-follicular cell 47
parathyroid ablation 126
– hormone 126
pathological classification 47, 102, 112
pentagastrin, stimulation of calcitonin 63
phaeochromocytoma 8, 52, 97
physiological control 37
pituitary hormones 34, 58
pleural metastases 90
podophyllotoxin 127, 135
procarbazine 127
profile scanning 80
prognosis 107, 129
–, papillary carcinoma and thyroiditis 56
prognostic index 129, 133
propanolol 125
protein bound ^{131}I 80

racial studies 8, 50
radiation hazards, see irradiation
– myelitis 116
– pulmonary fibrosis 119
radiography 89
^{123}radioiodine 69, 70
^{125}radioiodine 69
^{131}radioiodine 69
radioiodine therapy 110f.
– –, cause of cancer 14, 29
– – in management 37, 116
radiological protection 29
radio-nuclide imaging 66
radiotherapy 112f.
–, anaplastic carcinoma 119
–, complications 98, 116
–, external beam irradiation 115
–, follicular carcinoma 114
–, malignant lymphoma 121
–, medullary carcinoma 121
–, radioiodine 117
–, results 130
replacement therapy 125
reticulum-cell sarcoma 109
risk coefficient 27
– –, perspective 136
Rongelap Islanders 15

sarcoma 109
scanning 66
–, improved uptake 75
–, programme 74, 134
secondary tumors 35, 109
^{75}selenomethionine 73
sex, incidence 102
–, specific mortality rates 2
–,– survival rates 131
small cell carcinoma 48
solitary nodule 31, 65, 70
– –, investigation 72
– –, management 107, 110
– –, pathology 107
spindle-cell tumors 120
suppression therapy 125
surgery, anaplastic carcinoma 107
–, complications 108
–, follicular carcinoma 107
–, malignant lymphoma 107
–, management 102f.

–, medullary carcinoma 109
–, papillary carcinoma 108
–, results 130
–, solitary nodule 107
survival rates 129
– – by age 130
– – histology 131
– – by sex 130
– – by stage 131

^{99}technetium 69
teratoma, malignant 109
thermography 88
thiouracil, causing cancer 34
thymic irradiation 10, 28, 49
thyroglobulin antibodies 57
– assay 73, 82, 134
– – in benign adenoma 135
– – in well differentiated carcinoma 135
Thyroid Co-operative Group (EORTC) 129
thyroid nodule, cold 9
– –, hot 9
– –, solitary 9
– scan 69
– –, profile 43, 80
thyroiditis, auto-immune 9, 35, 52, 56
– and carcinoma 49, 56
–, chronic 4, 49
–, Hashimoto's 9, 35, 52, 56
– and lymphoma 58
thyrotoxicosis, see hyperthyroidism
thyroxine 34, 110, 114, 125

tinea capitis 28, 49
TRH assay 39, 126
– test 70, 114
tri-iodothyronine 125
TSAb 58
TSH 39, 57
–, assay 125
– and thyroid cancer 13
–, stimulation 39
–, – of tumor 40, 117
–, – of uptake 108
–, suppression 39
tumour markers, see biochemical markers

ultrasonography 87
undifferentiated carcinoma, causation 24
– –, management 108, 119
– –, pathology 47, 50
– –, results 120, 131
Utirik Islanders 26

vinblastine 127
vincristine 120
viral transformation 51
vitamin D 52, 126

well-differentiated carcinoma 134
– –, causation 9f., 24
– –, management 108, 113, 125
– –, markers 134
– –, pathology 50
– –, results 115, 131

Recent Results in Cancer Research

Sponsored by the Swiss League against Cancer. Editor in Chief: P. Rentchnick, Genève

For information about Vols. 1–9, please contact your bookseller or Springer-Verlag

10 NELSON, R. S.: Radioactive Phosphorus in the Diagnosis of Gastrointestinal Cancer.
11 FREEMAN, R. G. and J. M. KNOX: Treatment of Skin Cancer.
12 LYNCH, H. T.: Hereditary Factors in Carcinoma.
13 Tumours in Children, 2nd Edition. Edited by H. B. MARSDEN and J. K. STEWARD.
14 ODARTCHENKO, N.: Production Cellulaire Erythropoïétique.
15 SOKOLOFF, B.: Carcinoid and Serotonin.
16 JACOBS, M. L.: Malignant Lymphomas and Their Management.
17 Normal and Malignant Cell Growth. Edited by R. J. M. FRY, M. L. GRIEM, and W. H. KIRSTEN (Symposium).
18 ANGLESIO, E.: The Treatment of Hodgkin's Disease.
19 BANNASCH, P.: The Cytoplasm of Hepatocytes during Carcinogenesis. Electron- and Lightmicroscopical Investigations of the Nitrosomorpholineintoxicated Rat Liver.
20 Rubidomycin. A new Agent against Cancer. Edited by J. BERNARD, R. PAUL, M. BOIRON, C. JACQUILLAT, and R. MARAL.
21 Scientific Basis of Cancer Chemotherapy. Edited by G. MATHÉ (Symposium).
22 KOLDOVSKÝ, P.: Tumor Specific Transplantation Antigen.
23 FUCHS, W. A., J. W. Davidson, and H. W. FISCHER: Lymphography in Cancer. With contributions by G. JANTET and H. RÖSLER.
24 HAYWARD, J.: Hormones und Human Breast Cancer. An Account of 15 Years Study.
25 ROY-BURMAN, P.: Analogues of Nucleic Acid Components. Mechanisms of Action.
26 Tumors of the Liver. Edited by G. T. PACK and A. H. ISLAMI.
27 SZYMENDERA, J.: Bone Mineral Metabolism in Cancer.
28 MEEK, E. S.: Antitumour and Antiviral Substances of Natural Origin.
29 Aseptic Environments and Cancer Treatment. Edited by G. MATHÉ (Symposium).
30 Advances in the Treatment of Acute (Blastic) Leukemias. Edited by G. MATHÉ (Symposium).
31 DENOIX, P.: Treatment of Malignant Breast Tumors. Indications and Results.
32 NELSON, R. S.: Endoscopy in Gastric Cancer.
33 Experimental and Clinical Effects of L-Asparaginase. Edited by E. GRUNDMANN and H. F. OETTGEN (Symposium).
34 Chemistry and Biological Actions of 4-Nitroquinolin 1-Oxide. Edited by H. ENDO, T. ONO, and T. SUGIMURA.
35 PENN, I.: Malignant Tumors in Organ Transplant Recipients.
36 Current Concepts in the Management of Lymphoma and Leukemia. Edited by J. E. ULTMANN, M. L. GRIEM, W. H. KIRSTEN, and R. W. WISSLER (Symposium).
37 CHIAPPA, S., R. MUSUMECI, and C. USLENGHI: Endolymphatic Radiotherapy in Malignant Lymphomas. With contributions by G. BONADONNA, B. DAMASCELLI, G. FAVA, F. PIZZETTI, U. VERONESI.
38 KOLLER, P. C.: The Role of Chromosomes in Cancer Biology.
39 Current Problems in the Epidemiology of Cancer and Lymphomas. Edited by E. GRUNDMANN and H. TULINIUS (Symposium).
40 LANGLEY, F. A. and A. C. CROMPTON: Epithelial Abnormalities of the Cervix Uteri.
41 Tumours in a Tropical Country. A Survey of Uganda (1964–1968). Edited by A. C. TEMPLETON.
42 Breast Cancer: A Challenging Problem. Edited by M. L. GRIEM, E. V. JENSEN, J. E. ULTMANN, and R. W. WISSLER (Symposium).
43 Nomenclature, Methodology and Results of Clinical Trials in Acute Leukemias. Edited by G. MATHÉ, P. POUILLART, L. SCHWARZENBERG (Symposium).
44 Special Topics in Carcinogenesis. Edited by E. GRUNDMANN (Symposium).
45 KOLDOVSKÝ, P.: Carcinoembryonic Antigens.
46 Diagnosis and Therapy of Malignant Lymphoma. Edited by K. MUSSHOFF (Symposium).
47 Investigation and Stimulation of Immunity in Cancer Patients. Edited by G. MATHÉ and R. WEINER (Symposium).
48 Platinum Coordination Complexes in Cancer Chemotherapy. Edited by T. A. CONNORS and J. J. ROBERTS (Symposium).
49 Complications of Cancer Chemotherapy. Edited by G. MATHÉ and R. K. OLDHAM (Symposium).
50 Cancer Registry, Edited by E. GRUNDMANN and E. PEDERSEN (Symposium).

51 Gliomas. Current Concepts in Biology, Diagnosis and Therapy. Edited by J. HEKMATPANAH (Symposium).
52 The Ambivalence of Cytostatic Therapy. Edited by E. GRUNDMANN and R. GROSS (Symposium).
53 A. CLARYSSE, Y. KENIS, and G. MATHÉ: Cancer Chemotherapy.
54 Malignant Bone Tumors. Edited by E. GRUNDMANN.
55 MATHÉ, G.: Cancer Active Immunotherapy, Immunoprophylaxis, and Immunorestoration.
56 Lymphocytes, Macrophages, and Cancer. Edited by G. MATHÉ, I. FLORENTIN, and M.-C. SIMMLER (Symposium).
57 Breast Cancer: A Multidisciplinary Approach. Edited by G. ST. ARNEAULT, P. BAND, and L. ISRAËL (Symposium).
58 B. S. SCHOENBERG: Multiple Primary Malignant Neoplasms.
59 Selective Heat Sensitivity of Cancer Cells. Edited by A. ROSSI-FANELLI, R. CAVALIERE, B. MONDOVI, and G. MORICCA.
60 Tumors of the Male Genital System. Edited by E. GRUNDMANN and W. VAHLENSIECK (Symposium).
61 D. METCALF: Hemopoietic Colonies.
62 Tactics and Strategy in Cancer Treatment. Edited by G. MATHÉ (Symposium).
63 Antitumor Antibiotics. Edited by S. K. CARTER, H. UMEZAWA, J. DOUROS, and Y. SAKURAI (Symposium).
64 Lymphoid Neoplasias I: Classification, Categorization, Natural History.
65 Lymphoid Neoplasias II: Clinical and Therapeutic Aspects.
Lymphoid Neoplasias I & II. Proceedings of the 1977 CNRS-EORTC International Colloquium. Editors: G. MATHÉ, M. SELIGMANN, M. TUBIANA. Devided into two volumes.
66 Carcinogenic Hormones. Edited by C. H. LINGEMAN.
67/68 Adjuvant Therapies and Markers of Post-Surgical Minimal Residual Disease I & II. Proceedings of the 1978 Annual Plenary Meeting of the EORTC. Editors: G. BONADONNA, G. MATHÉ, S. E. SALMON. Divided into two volumes.
67 Markers and General Problems of Cancer Adjuvant Therapies.
68 Adjuvant Therapies of the Various Primary Tumors.
69 Strategies in Clinical Hematology. Edited by R. GROSS and K.-P. HELLRIEGEL.
70 New Anticancer Drugs. Edited by S. K. CARTER
71 Endocrine Treatment of Breast Cancer. Edited by B. HENNINGSEN, F. LINDER, C. STREICHELE.
72 CAWLEY, J. C., BURNS, G. F., HAYHOE, F. G. J.: Hairy-Cell Leukaemia.
73 Thyroid Cancer. Edited by W. DUNCAN.

MIX
Papier aus verantwortungsvollen Quellen
Paper from responsible sources
FSC® C105338

If you have any concerns about our products,
you can contact us on
ProductSafety@springernature.com

In case Publisher is established outside the EU,
the EU authorized representative is:
Springer Nature Customer Service Center GmbH
Europaplatz 3, 69115 Heidelberg, Germany

Printed by Libri Plureos GmbH
in Hamburg, Germany